CAREGIVING

An Errand of the Heart

Survival Tips for Caregivers

CAREGIVING

An Errand of the Heart

Survival Tips for Caregivers

by
Marguerite Mauss Eliason

with
Susan Chieko Eliason

Covenant Communications, Inc.

Published by Covenant Communications, Inc.
American Fork, Utah

Printed in the United States of America
First Printing: August 1995
01 00 99 98 97 96 95 94 10 9 8 7 6 5 4 3 2 1

Library of Congress Cataloging-in-Publication Data

Eliason, Marguerite M., 1930-
    Caregiving: an errand of the heart/by Marguerite M. Eliason, with Susan Chieko
        Eliason.
    p. cm.
    ISBN 1-55503-839-5
    1. Care of the sick. 2. Caregivers. I. Eliason, Susan Chieko. II. Title.
    R726.5.E39 1995
    362.1--dc20   95-21010
                                                                      CIP

Acknowledgments

My deepest gratitude—

to my family, who supported me, and to my parents, who gave me love and the opportunity to learn so much.

to the fine editors at Covenant—Helen Dixon, Valerie Holladay, and JoAnn Jolley.

to Carol Lynn Pearson, for allowing me to use her inspiring poem.

to my friends and associates who read the manuscript and offered their suggestions—Wayne Bush, George Durrant, Mary Ellen Edmunds, and Scott Peterson.

and to the caregivers who contributed their experiences to this book—Anne, Carol Lynn, Cheryl, Heather, Henry, Jennifer, Joan, Lynn, Lois, Martina, MaryDee, Marj, Mary Ellen, Phillip, Phyllis, Rachelle, Valerie, and Vivian—as well as countless others who shared of their time and hearts.

Dedication

Dedicated to my patient and loving husband, LeGrande, to whom I am happily heartbound forever.

Contents

TO AN AGED PARENT

by Carol Lynn Pearson

"Here, Dad—
Let's tuck in the napkin,
Just in case."

    The spoon makes its
    Hazardous trip to your mouth,
    And you glance at my face
    To see if I notice.

"All clean?"
Grab hold, then—up you come."

    I dry your body from the bath
    And tell of things I saw downtown
    To turn your mind from modesty.

"Now, if you need something
Just ring the bell.
I'll leave the door a little open
And turn on the hall light.
Good night."

    You close your eyes
    And curl into privacy,
    Free from the indignities of the day.
    "Sister, don't ever grow old,"
    You used to say.
    And here you are.

    Oh, Daddy, Daddy—
    There's no way to stop it
    Or to slow it.
    Let's just let it be.

    Time's strange circle
    Has brought around your turn
    To be comforted, and cleaned,
    And nursed.
    Shhhhhhh—It's all right.
    Let me hold you warm
    In your last days,
    As you did me in my first.

Preface

January, 1978. That was the month Mother had her first stroke. No one would have predicted she would be with us for another ten years. Nor did we realize then that Dad's annoying but seemingly minor skin irritation would blossom into a rare cancer, which manifested itself initially on the exterior, only later to turn inward—*so slowly*—to attack vital organs.

No, I didn't realize then that my parents would need care for some fourteen years. A week here, a month there, was how it all began. I would travel two states away to care for them through this siege or that, never able to completely relax after I returned home following an "episode." At one point, they moved from California to be near our family in Utah, eliminating for a time the need for me to leave town to lend a hand. But climate and altitude—and, ultimately, *home*—beckoned, and they returned to California. They were fighters, though, as independent as they could be 'til the end; Dad, especially, insisted on doing all he could for both of them until Mother became seriously incapacitated.

Gradually, Dad's strength diminished. He had begun radiation therapy for the now-aggressive case of *micosis fungoides*, and was barely up to caring for himself—most of the time. Mother continued to suffer a series of minor strokes and had begun to require full-time attention. My husband and I, meanwhile, had been considering a move to California, an idea whose time had apparently come.

Although I spent several hours every day at my parents'

home, we maintained separate households for some five years. Mother and Dad wanted to be self-sufficient as long as possible; we, likewise, valued privacy and relative autonomy. But when the time came to invite them to move into our home with us, they knew it was right. We knew it, too.

Such an experience it was! A blessed blur of foot rubs and sing-alongs, laundry by the truckload, precious reminiscences over yellowed photo albums, tapioca pudding with bing cherries, anguish when breath came haltingly at 3 a.m., and a nonstop four-generation carnival when our daughter and her family arrived for a stay of unknown duration. "You ought to write a book!" a friend exclaimed one day, as she watched the juggling act in disbelief from her front-row seat at our kitchen table.

I accepted the challenge—and promptly turned it over to my daughter Susan, without whom this book would never have been written.[1]

---

[1]See Author's Note at the end of this book.

Introduction

As a nation, we're living longer, healthier lives now than people have at any other period in history. Retirement communities are thriving, and in their wake a host of related amenities to support a lifestyle unheard of in more distant generations. "Seniors," as they're known, are wooed by travel agents, magazine publishers, time-share condominium developers, and dining establishments, to name just a few. And they're eating it up—they, who in times not so distantly past, would think twice before investing in econo-size Geritol!

With increasing longevity, however, is often seen the unfortunate concomitant of prolonged physical or mental deterioration. Paradoxically, the medical and technological advances that keep us alive and well can also keep us alive and not so well—and, as the courts will attest, sometimes just *alive*. Where do people go when the fun stops but life goes on?

Nursing homes, convalescent centers, pricey retirement villages with meals and maid service and a doctor on call—these and endless variations on similar themes exist to meet the needs of the declining elderly. There are those, of course, who choose to remain in their own homes as long as humanly possible, suffering the rigors and fears of isolation, age, and illness.

Then there's the semi-traditional alternative of moving in with relatives—usually children and their families. Many Asian cultures find nothing odd about this, a practice entirely consistent with their reverence for age and respect for parents who, in their view, gave all "up front" and are due to collect from the next generation on the other end. Alas, Eastern logic—and much of it is logical—doesn't always prevail on this hemisphere.[2]

But was it *logic*, after all, that prompted my husband and me to care for my parents the way we did? No, the mental processes didn't enter much into our decision at all. The invitation came from the *feeling* part of ourselves, the heart by which we were—and will always be—connected to these beloved ones. When frailty and disease rendered Mother and Father homebound, we responded from a purely emotional base. We were, you might say, *heart*bound.

The suggestions I offer in this book are intended to help you bridge heart and mind as you confront *your* caring challenge. One cannot operate forever—productively—from a feeling level; the head with all its rational cautions must enter at some point. You will notice that much of my advice is offered retrospectively, i.e., "Here's what I'd do if I had another chance." (As my granddaughter, Angela, used to say: "That's how you *don't* do it!") If there is wisdom to be learned from the errors of another, I readily confess that you will learn much from me.

No, this is not intended to be the all-inclusive last word on the subject of home health care. Relatively little of this book, in fact, explores the details and dynamics of day-in, day-out *physical* support; you'll find, instead, a broader, more philosophical tone in my reflections, and an emphasis on meeting the social and emotional needs of your aging loved one. You'll observe, too, a distinct leaning toward enhancing *your* well-being as caregiver.

And this work is short in length, easily read by most in one

[2] Worth noting, however, is the current (1995) estimate that, at any given time, only between five and twenty percent of older Americans make their home in an institutional care facility. The vast majority in need of care rely on family and friends for assistance.

or two sittings. It is designed for those whose reading time is limited but who need a word of encouragement, perhaps a little empathy, and some initial direction in the moment of crisis. Excellent written, audiovisual, and human resources exist to answer your specific questions on supporting the elderly, the mechanics of home care, helping your parents create a living will, and related issues. I refer to just a few of these at the end of the book; you will find no shortage of such information in public libraries, bookstores, hospital information centers, and community support groups. I encourage you to make yourself familiar with every potentially helpful resource, whether or not you think you need it now. The day may come when you'll be glad you know where to turn for help in a hurry.

A final disclaimer: Although I've tried to bring some balance to this effort by including selected observations and experiences of others in the caregiving role (past or present),[3] most of the contents of this book reflect *our family's* experience in the care of my parents—that which worked, as well as that which didn't work so well. Your circumstances will probably differ considerably; your desires to care for aging loved ones, for example, may exceed your capacity to do so. You may need to resolve certain emotional or relationship issues before you can embark on the caring journey with sufficient love and *for the right reasons.* Or, you may be feeling guilt—misplaced or legitimate—because you *could* be more involved in the care of loved ones than you now choose to be. You might be looking after a child or young adult whose physical and emotional needs are considerably different from those of an older patient.

In short, we come to our challenges from any number of backgrounds, and with a variety of attitudes and needs. What

---

[3] These I have placed throughout the book, some of which follow the heading "In the Words of Another." In consideration of their candor, my sources remain relatively anonymous, credited by first name only.

my husband and I tried to do, as primary caregivers for my parents in their declining years, may not be the best strategy for you. But as you read, try to look beyond practice into principle, and create applications for your situation.

Ultimately, all you and I may share is deep caring for those we love. And that is enough to keep us bound to beloved ones—heart and mind—forever.

PART I.

Making the Caring Decision

I was five years old when my father became disabled. A series of heart-related problems and strokes brought about a gradual deterioration in his condition that ended with his peaceful death in a rented hospital bed in our living room fourteen years later. I helped out all I could, but Mom was unquestionably the primary caregiver, a role she threw herself into almost obsessively. By the end, taking care of my Dad was her entire life, so his death was even more devastating than it might otherwise have been.

There was a sort of purity in Mom's role as caregiver. When sacrifice was necessary, she gave all. She suffered and agonized wholeheartedly. When Dad died, she lost everything and grieved fully. As with all sacrifices, however, there were some blessings, namely this: Her grief passed more quickly for her purity, and she recovered fully, creating a more full and independent life for herself than I could ever have imagined.

Not long after Dad died, Mom said something that I believe gave great insight into her attitude. It also provided me with a valuable lesson on peace of mind, a lesson I've never forgotten. When I remarked about the terrible toll caring for Dad had taken on her, Mom replied, "It was hard, but there's one thing I can honestly say: I don't have any regrets. No matter what anyone else might say or think, I know in my heart that I did everything for him I could. I'll never have to feel guilty."

—Phillip

Who Cares—and When, and Where?

By now, you know how my husband and I came to care for my parents—in their home and, finally, in ours—for just over fourteen years. Exactly when and how you meet your moment of choice is not as important as what you do about it. And *what* you do is usually a function of *who* will do. Are you the one most suited to care for an infirm relative or, from a practical point of view, is there someone else in the family whose time and circumstances suggest a more convenient arrangement? Should you consider sharing the care of Mother, Father, Grampy, or Aunt Myrtle with able siblings or cousins? Or do you think the loved one would fare better in a residential care facility or a nursing home, than in—

- a loving but cramped, noisy, cluttered household;

- a beautiful, well-appointed home with people who can't or don't want to deal with a homebound relative;

- an adequate home environment inhabited by good intentions but fueled with neglect; or

- a combination of any of the above?

We may be getting a little ahead of ourselves here. Let's assume, for the moment, that you face (or soon expect to encounter) the challenge of managing the care of an aging, and possibly bedridden or ill, loved one. Some even more basic questions for you first:

- How independent is Mother (or Father, or whoever) right now—physically, financially, and socially? Can she prepare her own meals, launder her clothes, keep her living environment clean? Is her income predictable and sufficient to meet her needs? Does she visit or welcome friends regularly, take part in community and social activities, enjoy a hobby or two? From your observations and those of other prospective caregivers in this situation, how much external help is really needed right now—and are you able to answer that question objectively?

- Why are *you* planning the care of a loved one (or engaged in the caring process already)? In the case of parent care, for instance, are you the oldest child? the only child? the "responsible one?" the dutiful daughter? the responsible namesake-son? the one without a full-time job? the one with a spare bedroom? the one *expected* to take on the project? Which brings us to the next question or, perhaps, note of caution:

- Could there be a touch (or more) of codependency factoring into the care equation? In other words, do you *need* to take responsibility for a major portion of a loved one's care in order to feel validated, useful, worthy, and *good?* (If you take time to think that one through and decide to answer affirmatively, hats off to you. Many would be offended at the question and deny vehemently the possibility that they could be influenced by other than altruistic motives.) On the other hand, is there a chance that your loved one could be trying to manipulate you into providing care that is either (a) not needed yet, or (b) beyond your capacity to give right now (or ever)? An otherwise benevolent soul can be highly skilled at cooking up an old family recipe heavily seasoned with guilt. Ominous overtones aside…

- What does the relative have to say? Is he or she capable of deciding on the best course of action? Does he or she *want to* leave home (or the current living arrangement)?

- If your loved one in need, you, or your support system—usually your immediate and extended family—decide after careful deliberation that external assistance is truly called for at this time, is moving the loved one out of his or her home the answer? Or can help be taken periodically into the home, for a while longer at least? If the loved one wants to remain at home but cannot afford to retain a full-time nurse or attendant, would hiring *part-time* help be a possibility? If his or her financial resources are lacking, can family members contribute regularly toward the cost of maintaining moderate in-home care (or perform needed services themselves on a rotation basis)?

- Finances permitting, would an infirm loved one prefer to move to a minimal care, home-like facility where meals, laundry, limited medical assistance, and a daily check ("alive and breathing") are included in a monthly charge? It may come as a surprise to some to learn that Uncle Roger really doesn't want to make a closet-sized, needs-paint den his new home. The same applies to the seriously ill or bedridden patient needing more comprehensive care. She, too, may prefer to live somewhere other than with a relative. Discuss with your loved one—as honestly and kindly as possible—what he or she needs and wants, and what you are able, *realistically,* to provide. Do not assume the role of problem solver; make the care decision *together.*

If at first inquiry it appears that the idea of bringing the loved one into your home—or otherwise accepting major responsibility for his or her care—is worthy of further exploration, consider *these* questions:

- Do you have (or can you arrange) the space, furniture, and other physical resources for your guest? For that matter, will you consider him or her a "guest," or are you prepared to welcome a new member of the family to your home?

- Are you in a position to offer the kind of care you may want to provide, in or out of your home? Do you have the time, physical stamina, and emotional and financial resources that will be required? What are your assets and limitations, tangible and intangible? Exceeding your limits exacts a toll you may be unable to pay.

- If you (or you and your spouse) work outside the home, have you considered who will care for the loved one during those hours? how he or she will spend time in your absence? what he or she will do when you are absent for extended periods, e.g., vacations and business trips?

- How do you handle change and stressful situations? How well do you cope with new demands? How far will your "emotional tether" stretch to meet increasing demands as your loved one becomes more dependent?

- If you have a family of your own, how far can you extend yourself beyond your more fundamental obligations? How supportive are your spouse and children? What will they be asked to sacrifice or contribute? Will your children be required to give up a private bedroom, for instance? Are they willing to render service or complete daily chores to assist you in your role as primary caregiver? Will you be required to contribute financially in such a way that will seriously limit your ability to meet your children's needs? *Are you and your spouse and children comfortable with the new roles you will assume?*

- Has a living will been prepared, if desired, and a power of attorney executed that will remain in effect should the loved one become mentally incapacitated?

You're getting the idea. Rarely is there a simple solution, a well-lit path defining an obvious course. Add to the foregoing a list of your own questions, and invest the time you need to respond to them completely and honestly. *Discuss and write them out*—concerns, options, restraints, considerations, and personal desires—in complete detail. Again, involve your loved one, to the extent he or she is able: What does he or she want to have happen? How do his or her needs and desires correspond with *your* inclinations and resources?

When you've done your homework, you may conclude that (a) this is not the time, (b) you're not the one, (c) an outside care facility would be the most prudent choice, (d) "no help needed, thank you," or (e) any combination or variation of the above, which eliminates you from the caregiver role at the moment.

If, however, after sufficient thought and consultation with all parties concerned, you decide to embrace the role of primary or assistant caregiver, the rest of what follows is for you. Not everything is here for you, by any means; this is just the beginning of what you'll learn in the process of providing support for someone you love and taking care of *yourself*.

A Care-Full Start: Merging Expectations

Overheard in Household A:

> *Of course Mother's not here! I thought you were picking her up at the beauty salon.... Sure I know what time it is.... What little green pill?*

...and in Household B:

> *Papa Bob likes to do* what *with his social security check?! In my entire life, I've never been to the races, and here we are, sharing our beans and franks, and the bedroom we don't have, and....*

Won't do much for a marriage, will it? Not to mention that Mother's newly coiffed head may be in serious pain because she didn't get her green pill on time.

Virtually all conflict—in any relationship, any situation—results from mismatched expectations and different (and often unspoken) agendas. When hearts and minds agree that a major sharing and caring time has arrived (e.g., Father moves into your home, or you assume heavier responsibility for his health and well-being), the first order of business is to call a joint session of the house, followed by frequent and regular subcommittee meetings.

And who are the attendees?

If you're married, you and your spouse meet together first—alone. What do you both need to have happen in order to continue to provide the care you have agreed to give? Is sharing or rotating caring tasks daily, weekly, monthly, *actually going to work?* What elements of your current lifestyle will be adjusted to accommodate your new caring roles? *Do not* simply assume that it will be "business as usual" with an exception here or there.

Next comes the family meeting. Ideally, this occurs on two levels—with *your* siblings, especially those who are close enough to share the care of a parent (if it's a parent in need), and with members of your immediate household (most likely, a spouse and children). You've thought about these questions before inviting your loved one to share your home, but consider them once more:

- To what extent can your brothers and sisters in the area assist with parent care when you have obligations outside the home? For example, can they provide rides to doctor appointments, senior social events, shopping, etc.?

- What sacrifices will your spouse and children need to make?

- Will you have considerably less leisure time to spend with your spouse, for instance, and how can you both compensate for the loss of frequent shared activity (if such indeed has been part of your life to this point)?

- Will your children need to look elsewhere for help with homework, and will they be asked to give more—a bedroom, perhaps—for the indefinite future?

- Can you help your children identify concrete and regular opportunities to assist in the caring process, and thereby feel more a part of the effort?

Worth noting is that such family meetings are not one-time events. You will want to schedule regular get-togethers with siblings and your immediate household to discuss what's working well and what isn't, reallocate workloads, and consider alternative care arrangements if the current system needs an adjustment.

A brief "time out" before continuing this discussion: If you read the first chapter in this section carefully, you'll recognize that these detailed spouse and family gatherings are actually *second*-round meetings. Before deciding to involve yourselves more extensively in the caring process, you answered the questions in the previous section (and more, I hope, of your own creation), individually and with available siblings, spouse, and children. At this point, the issue is not "Shall we care for the loved one?" but "*How* can we provide the day-to-day care we have decided to give?" Making service assignments or requesting any kind of sacrifice from family members can be counterproductive and perceived as manipulative, if not preceded by explicit agreement that opening heart (and possibly home) is truly what the family is willing to do.

Your Ideas:

-

-

-

PART II.
Caring for the Caregiver(s)

So there I was, trying to manage menopause and hide the gray ("because I'm worth it"), soon to be reminded at every ticket counter and restaurant that I—horrors!—qualified for the senior citizen rate, when I found myself in an awkward position: playing junior fiddle to the senior senior-citizen set. While I never stopped learning from my parents and feeling their moral and emotional strength, our roles shifted rather abruptly the day Mother had her first stroke. Suddenly, I was feeding, bathing, nurturing, parenting a parent. Life would never be the same.

My friend, Marj, put it well as she reflected on her experience: "To be an effective parent to either the young or the old means coming to terms with your own childhood past. To become a parent to your parent seems especially difficult, partly so because you now become the 'responsible one,' and the fiction that your parent will somehow always be there for you is all played out. You, the caregiver, also need to deal with the realization that not only will your parent move on, but so will you."

It's easy, I suppose, to look back at what I could have done to better manage my own health and meet personal needs as I took care of my parents. I don't regret for a moment my investment in their health and comfort, but that doesn't mean I wouldn't have done a few things differently, given the clearer perspective of hindsight. To anyone in the position of primary caregiver, I offer the following pages.

Coping and the Fine Art of Temporary Escape

In the words of a current caregiver...

> *One Sunday I heard a woman speak at church on the experience of caring for her elderly mother. Her mother had already died, so the comments were in the past tense—and heavily flavored with sweet reflections. Deep in the middle of my own caregiving season now, I should have found the presentation comforting, illuminating, encouraging, or otherwise helpful in some way. Instead, I went home and straight to bed. And it was only 10 o'clock in the morning.*
>
> —Valerie

Caring for my parents was, at times, a joy. It was also demanding, frustrating, and occasionally downright exasperating. During those moments that I desperately needed a nap or a good meal, neither of which I perceived to be even a remote possibility in the foreseeable future, I would occasionally indulge in a healing mental departure, a flight of fancy you might say. I'm convinced that anyone who is feeling overwhelmed or confined—even by happy and willing choice—can benefit from checking out, albeit briefly, on the wings of liberating fantasy. More on that in a page or two.

Then there are times when a daydream simply won't do the trick. I feel I need to say that right up front so that what follows doesn't destroy my credibility entirely. You know by now that this is essentially an account of *my* caregiving experience, and my typical responses to stress may not be yours. And had I known *then* what I know *now*, I believe I would have allowed others to bear a greater measure of the responsibility that I assumed—even *absorbed*—without really thinking about it. I address that subject in a later chapter.

First, a word on following the more prudent road of well-managed self-care. My best advice: Put on *your* oxygen mask first! That's what they tell us in the friendly skies, in case cabin air gets thin. What good are we to others, after all, if we're dead or in a faint? That's why part two of this book precedes part three—or, why "care for the caring" comes before "care for the cared for." This means, simply, that *you* need to eat correctly, exercise, and get enough rest—and external support—to function well enough to help provide the same for another.

Easier said than done, I assure you. In retrospect, I would have taken better care of myself as I cared for my parents. One thing I *did* manage to do fairly well was make time for regular exercise on my stationary bicycle. I had knee surgery in the middle of our caring decade, and maintaining the use of my limbs meant a frequent physical workout. This required getting up at 5 a.m. to exercise, shower, and prepare for the day, which usually began for the needy vocal majority at six. Except during periods of intensity or crisis, I managed to log between ten and fifteen go-nowhere miles most mornings, which made *all* the difference in my ability to manage the stresses of the day with stamina and good humor.

So much for the self-congratulatory remarks. What I could have done better was adopt the healing nutrition I have subsequently embraced. Failure to take time for regular, balanced meals (or to eliminate excessive animal products and fat) no doubt contributed to the gallbladder disease and subsequent surgery that made its untimely entrance into my life during one of Mother's most critical seasons. While endless books on diet and fitness may exist, I submit that relatively few simple, trustworthy, *accurate* sources of information have been written on the subject. (See my recommendations in the Suggested Readings and Resources section at the end.) Why I have chosen to adopt a low-fat, high-fiber, low animal-product nutrition program—and what rewards this decision has already produced for me and my family—is a subject for another day, perhaps another book. For present purposes, let me just remind you that batteries don't run on aftershave, automobiles don't go anywhere on kerosene, and humans fail to thrive (or sometimes even survive) on sporadic or indulgent intakes of grease, flesh, and sugar. And you, fellow giver of care, need all the high-performance fuel you can get.

Okay, now for the fantasy I constructed to survive and even grin my way through the hardest times. Contributing to my sanity on those days was the creation of my alter ego, "Mrs. Jim Olson." Central to the character of Mrs. Olson was blessed anonymity. On those days I craved privacy and aloneness, those times when I wished no one knew my name, I would call my daughter, Susan, and whisper conspiratorially, "This is Mrs. Jim Olson. I've had it; I'm leaving. I'm on my way—but you know where you can find me."

Susan knew exactly what I meant.

So that *you'll* know, too, the story of Mrs. Jim Olson—in her own words—goes something like this:

> *If I ever end up missing, you'll find me in North Platte, Nebraska. In the diner located next to the Greyhound bus terminal, to be exact. I'll be the one in the tight pink polyester uniform, smiling blankly as I pour lukewarm coffee and serve doughnuts as glazed as the look in my eye.*
>
> *I'll be wearing a little name tag that says something like "Madge" or "Trudy"; for legal purposes, I'll be "Mrs. Jim Olson." (I picked that out years ago as the perfect no-frills, betcha-can't-find-me-again-as-hard-as-you-try name. I'm looking forward to trying it out.)*
>
> *Ah, the simple, anonymous life. How good it sounds to me sometimes. I really wouldn't trade my world right now, with all its glaring recognitions and ceaseless demands, because it consists mainly of people I love. Needy people, may I add, but people I cherish, nonetheless. I'm getting better at letting these dear folks do for them-*

selves what they can, which can be more trying than simply doing it myself. I mean, have you ever watched a pineapple-shaped ninety-one-year-old with high blood pressure tie his own shoelaces? an ignited, beanie-coptered six-year-old spread peanut butter on every-thing but bread as he makes his own lunch? Do you agree with me that sometimes it's just easier to let a curious, jam-besmeared tod-dler examine your fine bone china with sticky little hands than to deal with the high-decibel outcome of letting this child hear "no"?

It feels good to laugh, to see in new light the hilarities and incon-gruities of a four-generation household. I feel better already. I think I can handle this—for a bit longer, anyway. But while I'm in my right mind, let me just say again that this contentment may not last. My wick may fail to meet the wax one day, and I'll be gone. My absence will be noticeable, believe me, and no one will have a clue where I am. Except you. You'll know where to find me.

Lesson for you: *Check out* when you must; don't burn out. When you begin to feel physical symptoms of unrelieved stress—stomach disorders, headaches, inability to sleep—or you find yourself snapping at family and friends, or denying that you have a problem or need assistance, the time has come to seek relief. In many cases, a little more self-care (see Additional Suggestions below) and perhaps a restructuring of family responsibilities will meet your needs. If you sense that you're approaching your breaking point, however, you've passed the point of managing tension with a simple exercise in imagination or an afternoon matinee; in this case, you would be well-advised to consult a counselor, ecclesiastical leader, doctor, or a caregiver support group.

Additional Suggestions:

- Simplify, *simplify!* "Clear the decks" of every extraneous complication or even benign distraction. Release your-self—without guilt—from otherwise meaningful but time- and energy-consuming committees and benevolent obligations that threaten to compromise your sanity and health.[4] Extend the purge to your physical surroundings as well: ruthlessly discard or give away anything in your home or living area that clutters or fails to serve a useful purpose. Enlist the aid of your family in this ongoing simplification venture—certainly at the beginning of your caring challenge, especially if you need to rearrange living space to provide for a loved one. You'll be amazed at how much less complicated your world appears, increased responsibilities on the home-front notwithstanding, when you pare back to the essentials in every facet of life.[5]

- Take time daily to get away from the scene—alone. Sit under a tree for half an hour and meditate, or simply clear your head and think of nothing at all. Feed the ducks or pigeons at a nearby park, if that feeds *your* soul. At least once a week, break away to enjoy a therapeutic full-body massage, try a new hairstyle, or buy that dress you've been eyeing in the window of your favorite store. Far from frivolous indulgences, such small pleasures replenish diminishing reserves and enable you to maintain (or regain) much-needed *joie de vivre* and good humor.

- Take your spouse, child, or a friend to lunch. Order your favorite items from the menu, and spend at least an hour

---

[4] Consider this a worthwhile rule of thumb even when your caring duties are a thing of the past.

[5] If you need further incentive to simplify your life, take time to read *Gift from the Sea*, by Anne Morrow Lindbergh. Among the pearls in this short, quickly read book is this reminder: "It is not merely the trivial which clutters our lives but the important as well. We can have a surfeit of treasures—an excess of shells, where one or two would be significant" (Pantheon, New York, 1955, p. 115).

discussing anything and everything but your role as caregiver—unless, of course, that's what you *want* to talk about.

• Get some oxygen! Have you ever noticed that when you're stressed or absorbed in a task, you can virtually stop breathing? Not enough to cause unconsciousness or death, perhaps, but certainly enough to induce unnecessary fatigue and decreased vitality. Two simple and enormously rewarding treatments: First, develop the habit of consciously *thinking* about your breathing. Then, create a "breathing cue." When you hear or say the word *but,* for instance, take a deep breath through your nose, feeling your chest expand. Hold the breath for a few seconds, and then release it slowly through your mouth. You may want to accompany this cleansing ritual by gently turning your head from side to side, front to back, and consciously lowering your shoulders. Instant oxygen, instant tension release, instant refreshment! A second way to deliver healing oxygen to every cell of your body is to enjoy a brisk walk, or other form of aerobic exercise, as many days of the week as you possibly can. Even if you can no more than make it up and down your neighborhood sidewalk once or twice for only minutes at a time, do what you can, breathing deeply as you move. As I indicated earlier, I simply would not have survived this most challenging period of my life without greeting each morning from the seat of my stationary bicycle.

• Resist any reflexive tendencies toward excessive independence, and accept the assistance of those who offer to help. Doing so does *not* suggest character weakness, and will preserve your emotional and physical well-being.

- As frequently as your schedule will realistically permit, engage the caregiving services of a sibling or paid attendant, and plan a guilt-free afternoon or weekend retreat with your spouse or a good friend. But what if the very thought of escape makes you feel like Valerie?

> *While I do my best to provide for my mother's needs now that she's living with me, I simply have to get away occasionally and live a life of my own. It's hard, though. I went out with friends the other night, for instance, and before I left I made sure that Mom was comfortable and settled. But throughout the evening, I kept thinking to myself, "Mom would have enjoyed this restaurant so much. I should have brought her along."*

It's a natural response—but let it go. Think of it this way: By allowing yourself some needed diversion from time to time, you're essentially restoring your soul and improving your ability to better care for your loved one. You need not travel far to enjoy a day at a lake or beach, have a picnic in a mountain canyon, or otherwise surround yourself in a healing natural environment. Talk with your partner-in-escape about the life you plan to create when current obligations are no more. Planning for the future—while enjoying the moment—can enhance feelings of well-being (some say it actually increases your endorphin level), and help fuel the remainder of your caring journey.

- A rich spiritual life can contribute immeasurably to your peace and serenity, giving you added strength to cope when the burdens seem too heavy to bear. To me, this is an essential element of graceful survival under any challenging circumstance. I dedicate the next chapter to a brief treatment of the subject.

Your Ideas:

-

-

-

Spiritual Support and Serenity

Honour thy father and thy mother: that thy days may be long upon the land which the Lord thy God giveth thee. (Ex. 20:12.)

Frequent prayer, heartfelt communion with a compassionate Heavenly Father, carried me through the stormy moments, and helped me to view such times as the *moments* they truly were, when viewed from a more long-term perspective. Though my mother and father were my parents, they were God's children, and I sensed his appreciation for the care I provided to those he loved so much. I didn't always have the luxury of a formal prayer on bended knee; frequently, my heavenward petitions took place in silence as I navigated the freeway or waited in line at the grocery store.

Demanding schedule notwithstanding, I found further comfort and guidance from reading the scriptures regularly, if only a few verses at a time. Among my favorites during the most difficult days was this comforting invitation from the Savior:

> *Come unto me, all ye that labour and are heavy laden, and I will give you rest. Take my yoke upon you, and learn of me; for I am meek and lowly in heart: and ye shall find rest unto your souls. For my yoke is easy, and my burden is light. (Matt. 11:28-30.)*

And when I was exhausted, short on patience, or otherwise tempted to underestimate the impact of my demeanor on my parents, I recalled that "a merry heart doeth good like a medicine..." (Prov. 17:22).

As much as possible, I continued to participate regularly in formal worship services, finding comfort in reminders of the resurrection, and in the counsel of my bishop (my ecclesiastical leader) and trusted friends. On more than one occasion, I found myself sitting quite contentedly on a chapel pew, joining in song with the congregation and choir, when I'd feel the warmth of a hand on my shoulder. Then a simple, "How are you today, Peggy?" whispered in my ear—and the fatigue and frustration I'd held all week would spill down my cheeks and splash across the open pages of the hymnal on my lap. "It's going to get better," I'd reply, more surprised than embarrassed by my occasional reaction to the simplest gesture of love. *I need thee, O I need thee; every hour I need thee*—lines from a favorite hymn speaking a plea for divine aid, immersed more than once in a healing tide of tears.

Which brings me to this thought: I believe that the Savior, Jesus Christ, came not only to save us from our sins as I had once supposed, but also to bless us as we deal with *all* of life's vicissitudes. He is there to strengthen us in weakness and make us adequate where we are naturally inadequate. Never before in my life had I been made so forcefully aware of this truth than when I faced the daily certainty of a trial with an uncertain end. A trial I accepted, I *chose,* mind you, but an enormously challenging one, nonetheless. On those occasions when I knew that my strength was gone and I could simply do no more—when so much more was required—I turned to the Lord in silent prayer, and asked for help to manage the task at hand and gracefully survive the day. Like manna, a one-day (and sometimes, one-hour) supply of physical strength or emotional tether was mercifully extended, accompanied by a sense of peace and—this was most significant to me—a feeling of heavenly approval of my efforts to honor worthy parents.

In the words of another...

> When my mother became physically dependent on me, I was angry—angry at the situation that had thrown my life into such a tailspin and required me to make painful changes and sacrifices. I was also angry with Mother. She and I hadn't gotten along that well

in recent years, and now here she was in my home, requiring virtually every moment, spare and otherwise. I can't begin to describe the frustration and despair that characterized my response to spilled bowls of soup and soiled bedsheets; I began to believe that I must have offended God in some grievous way to deserve such punishment.

On the day my depression reached its peak, I found myself in a doctor's waiting room, idly scanning a Bible I'd found on the table in front of me. And then it happened: Words of the Apostle Paul jumped off the page and plunged squarely into my heart: "And though I bestow all my goods to feed the poor, and though I give my body to be burned [or, I thought, though I wear myself out and share limited resources with my mother who demands all I have and more], and have not charity, it profiteth me nothing. Charity suffereth long, and is kind...is not easily provoked, thinketh no evil; ...Beareth all things, believeth all things, hopeth all things, endureth all things. Charity never faileth..." (1 Cor. 13:3-8, emphasis added). Oh, how I needed the gift of charity!

I didn't wait until I returned home to ask God for the endowment I so desperately required; I silently poured out my heart as I sat on the plastic orange waiting-room couch, to the God who urges throughout all of scripture to "Ask, and it shall be given you; seek, and ye shall find; knock, and it shall be opened unto you" (Matt.7:7). Inaudibly yet with sincerity born of great need, I pleaded for love and greater patience.

God's generous and immediate response was no less real than if I had been presented with a physical gift. Suddenly, I recalled in visionary detail the mother of my childhood—that kind, warm, soft woman who had gradually taken on the harsh and critical demeanor of one who has known emotional distress and chronic illness. I remembered, for instance, the time she had gone without a much-needed pair of new work shoes so that I could be spared the embarrassment and discomfort of another winter in my thin brown coat. This was the mother who had worked two, sometimes three, jobs to support my sisters and me after Dad passed away without warning—and without life insurance—and still managed to sing us to sleep most nights.

Interrupting my reverie, the nurse announced that the doctor *was ready to see me. I rose from my seat, my eyes blurred with tears, but the weight on my shoulders considerably lightened. Now, several years after Mother's death, I can assure you that following the Biblical counsel to "cast thy burden upon the Lord" yields sweet rewards. Truly, "he [God] shall sustain thee" (Ps. 55:22)—and "charity never faileth" (1 Cor. 13:8).*

—Heather

Additional Suggestions:

- If I had it to do over, I'd keep a journal. Time may not have permitted frequent or extensive written revelation of my thoughts and feelings during the height of the caregiving period, but "now and then" would have been better than nothing. You may already recognize the therapeutic (to say nothing of historical) value of committing a record of your daily life to paper, in which case you need no persuasion from me. But if you haven't started keeping a personal history, *don't wait until life gets easier before you start!* To capture the intensity of life *as it happens* is to preserve the essence of life. And from my limited journal-keeping experience, I can tell you that it simply feels good to get it out.

  If you don't enjoy writing, try telling it to a tape recorder or, for the less inhibited, the video camcorder. You may even want to assemble a scrapbook, collecting photographs, pressed flowers, and other memorabilia representative of this chapter of your life. Invite other members of your family to contribute to this effort; make it a shared project in which you may all take pride and comfort.

- In a related vein, consider creating a file or notebook of uplifting and personally meaningful poems, scriptural passages, stories, and hymns, to which you can turn in particularly stressful hours. You may wish to collaborate with the patient in this particular endeavor, helping him or her contribute to and benefit from what can become a most reassuring resource.

Your Ideas:

-

-

-

PART III.
Caring for the Loved One

*"Pure religion and undefiled before God and the Father is this,
To visit the fatherless and widows in their affliction...." (James
1:27.)*

*We often have wondered how many older people there are who
have no one to rescue them from avoidable deterioration. How
many, exhibiting impaired mental behavior, are consigned to institu-
tions, where they are overtranquilized, brought to a feeling of use-
lessness, robbed of morale and dignity, finally diagnosed as
demented and written off to die in a human warehouse.*

—Hugh Downs[6]

*Personally, I felt a commitment to help both my mother and
father during their final days. It was more than simply a nice,
decent thing to do; the way I saw it, my parents helped me into this
life and it was my dutiful pleasure to help them out of it. Having said
that, I don't believe in the "at all costs" approach, either. If your circumstances don't permit you to do everything you'd like, don't feel
guilty. In my opinion, finding balance without guilt is the greatest
challenge of the whole process, and it's one that only each individual
involved can assess.*

—Anne

[6]"My Father's New Life," *Parade Magazine*, February 28, 1993.

Independence: An Attitude We Never (Want to) Outgrow

In the words of one whose mother suffers from Alzheimer's...

> *Mother packed all of her belongings in front of the door Friday evening, saying she was leaving for home early Saturday. Thinking we could make her forget about going home alone, my sister and I watched a video with Mother until late. Then I put her suitcases on one of the double beds and covered them with a blanket. Mother awoke earlier than we on Saturday, carried her boxes and suitcases downstairs to the front door, and came up demanding her car keys.*
>
> *"Wait until I bathe and make some phone calls," I suggested, "and then I'll drive you home."*
>
> *"Give me the keys," she retorted. "You're just stalling."*
>
> —Henry

My little granddaughter, Mariana, is not unwilling to accept a favor. She is, in fact, more than able to make her wants known to anyone in a position to oblige. Heaven help you, though, if you try to hurry things along by offering unwelcome assistance, i.e., doing for Mariana what she can—or, more accurately, *wants to*—do for herself, especially in the area of developing motor skills. Anyone who tries to get the buffet line moving a little faster by dishing up Mariana's peas, for instance, is in for thirty-one pounds of determined resistance, accompanied by this ear-splitting, abbreviated declaration of independence: "Can do it by *'self!*"

Independence. A coveted condition we as a nation struggled to acquire over two centuries ago, and a state of being we seek from our first babyish attempts at self-sufficiency. A gift, a *right*, we do not relinquish easily—and do not give up at all

36

unless forced by mental or physical incapacity or forfeited by violation of law.

I knew that, kind of, when I cut my father's meat at the dinner table, or rushed to comb mother's hair. I was just being helpful, I reasoned, and doing for them what was more of a challenge for them than for me. At times, they willingly accepted my efforts to spare any exertion or frustration on their part. On other occasions, however, I was confused by their resistance to my well-meaning—but, in retrospect, downright smothering—involvements in matters of personal care.

I don't think I'd do it again, given the chance. At least, I would think twice before rushing in to perform an act of personal service that could be interpreted as my belief that the recipient was not capable of handling that task himself. It might be hard at times, just as it is to watch a child's fumblings, when *my* schedule could be better accommodated by moving things along. How often, I have since wondered, were my unnecessary interventions conveniently cloaked in a costume of benevolence?

In at least one area, though, we did quite well—especially Dad. Until he became too ill to function, Dad got up and dressed, ate a hearty brunch (he didn't break any speed records getting things together in the morning), and toodled off to his downtown office, where he supervised operations and managed the books. Toward the end, his business activities consisted less of poring over columns with his rubber thumb and green visor, and more along the lines of ordering exotic marmalades, nut clusters, and pickled chili sauces from specialty catalogs for unsuspecting acquaintances. And visiting Juanita next door at the plant shop to see how her philodendrons were getting along. And rearranging the family photos under glass on his desk. Attired in his sprightliest garb, complete with the jaunty tweed fedora sporting an orange feather, Dad met each moment with aplomb. This was *his* little empire, and let no one forget it. Even when battling the ravages of radiation and chemotherapy, rarely did Mr. Mauss miss a morning managing minutiae! His business was his *raison d'être* which, along with his unfailing humor and relish for simple daily delights, propelled him well into his ninety-second year.

I'm so glad that Dad felt it more important to be "productive" than "pajama-ed" most mornings. Which brings me to thoughts of Mother, and those amazing escapades in the kitchen....

It was really quite a sight: There stood my eighty-three-year-old stroke-patient mother, who, although unable to attend to many of her basic needs, now stood hunched over the kitchen sink. Vegetable peeler in hand, she was attacking an innocent carrot with a vengeance. That the surrounding area was beginning to look like fallout from a minor holocaust did not matter; Mother was thick in the middle of a challenge that consumed her every faculty, and loving every shredding minute.

It could have been just another cleanup job for me, but I decided I'd much rather deal—happily—with the scattered remains of one of Mother's rare and consuming joys than maintain spotless order on the homefront. Mother spent many of her final days taking oxygen and sipping bland strawberry-flavored nourishment through a straw. But when she was able to "help," we gave her every opportunity. Here was the family matriarch, once queen of the kitchen (and of the classroom, stage, and choirloft), whose body had gradually refused to fulfill the demands of a high-performance agenda. Her willingness to serve, however, had not expired. An occasional stint in the kitchen peeling vegetables—or folding towels, or giving a short voice lesson—increased Mother's alertness and helped her retain her prime spot in the family mosaic.

In the words of a caregiving couple… First, from the wife:

Taking care of our parents in their later years can be a time for happiness, and a wonderful opportunity to repay them for the love and care they have given us. However, this happy time and time of repayment can have its challenges—even some anguish and tears.

Probably the most difficult time we faced was when we recognized that we had to become full-time, rather than part-time, caregivers for our parents. Helping our parents also come to that realization was an even greater challenge.

My husband says the hardest day of his life was when he had to tell his parents that it was no longer safe for Dad to drive his car. The dents and scratches on the car were visible evidence of Dad's physical and mental decline. Mom and Dad felt perfectly safe on the road, however, and did not believe that they were putting the safety of others at risk. After all, they drove slowly, didn't go far, and as for those dents and scratches—they were simply the inevitable outcome of leaving the car in parking lots.

Needless to say, it wasn't easy convincing Lynn's parents that the time had come to surrender the car keys. But with time, they came to realize that having their children chauffeur them wasn't all that bad. They even came to enjoy the door-to-door service we provided.

We don't have any magical solutions to offer—just some suggestions from our experience. For instance, we need to remember that being independent and feeling independent are two different things. Even when parents need our full-time care, we can help them feel independent. Also, having a positive attitude, not making parents feel like they're a burden, being patient and understanding, and expressing love often, will help parents maintain a sense of control over their lives even though we care increasingly for their needs.

—*Joan*

The following short piece, written by Joan's husband, Lynn, offers the words he feels his father would have used on the morning he surrendered his driving privileges:

Our son [Lynn], oh, how he wanted to obtain his license to drive a car! That license represented to him the status and independence he so much wanted—access to the world when and where he chose! And now it seems like only a few years later, he stands here in our family room a grown-up man but still the same young son to us, announcing that "after his careful consideration" we, his mother and father, should no longer have the same privilege that not long ago we gave to him—the right to drive our own car. Surrendering this last symbol of life and independence, even the freedom to go to the store when we want, we wonder what on earth is left for us.

Yes, there is pain and anxiety in our son's eyes. In words we don't want to hear, he again promises to take care of our needs, to be a good son, and to seek only our happiness and well-being.

But the truth of the matter is that this is the darkest morning of our lives, and we are certain it is the same for our son.

—Lynn

Additional Suggestions:

- As appropriate, discuss decisions that affect your loved one in areas large and small. Elicit his or her input regarding who might be invited to Sunday dinner, what traditions to highlight during the holidays, how to redecorate the family room.

In the words of another…

I suggest that you involve the patient in every possible decision in which he or she is capable of participating. For example, we asked the Meals on Wheels organization to provide lunch for my somewhat frail mother who lives alone. A well-meaning relative contacted the service and requested that Mother be served low-fat, no-salt meals. Mother complained, saying that the food was also "no-flavor"—and then she changed the order on her own. The more health-conscious meals would have been the relative's choice, but not my mother's. Since Mother was still of sound mind, and aware of and willing to accept consequences for her decisions, compliance with a restrictive diet should have been her choice—no matter what the medical indications.

—Marj

- When Mother or Dad could join us at the table for family meals, we frequently invited one or the other to offer a blessing on the food. Dad, especially, enjoyed participating in routine and celebratory family activities, and would often ask one of us to drive him to the local bakery where he would select a lemon pie or some other treat to contribute to the festivities.

- Besides inviting your willing patient to peel carrots or shell peas, why not also enlist help rocking the baby or reading to a toddler? stamping envelopes? wrapping gifts? Add to the list other small chores your loved one is capable of performing. Unless she or he wants to be alone, your patient should be encouraged to undertake such tasks in the family room or wherever the action is. Half the fun is working together!

- Recognize that not every patient covets independence and autonomy; you may find yourself caring for one who will go to some lengths to persuade you that his or her care or responsibilities belong upon your shoulders. Should you observe this tendency in any of its subtle (and not-so-subtle) manifestations, explain in gentle but frank terms what you can and cannot do to assist. Make sure, of course, that your conclusions are valid and based on repeated observation and discussion. You may discover that your loved one is simply lonely; what appear to be unreasonable demands for your assistance may be no more than thinly veiled requests for more time spent in conversation and camaraderie.

Your Ideas:

-
-
-

Privacy and Parades: Accommodating Needs for Space

Mother had the master bed and bath, and things couldn't have worked out better—for all of us. It was a small sacrifice, really, considering that she spent most of her day in semi-confinement (the largest, sunniest bedroom was the nicest place to be) and that she frequently needed immediate access to bathroom facilities. While this may not be a workable option for most other families in similar circumstances, the larger principle here should apply across the board: Making the patient as comfortable as possible—and her care as convenient as circumstances will allow—should prove to be well worth it in the long haul. If her mobility is not a problem, you may not need to consider forfeiting your bedroom even temporarily as you arrange her accommodations.

Had we not been able, for one reason or another, to provide such user-friendly arrangements for Mother, we would still have included one essential feature next to her bed: the Drawer. In the Drawer, Mother kept her cache of sweets and other top-secret (but not life-threatening) contraband. Mother, who in her better days served homemade lima bean bisque and sent Dad out to buy stoneground, salt-free, whole-wheat bread available only at the inconveniently located health-food store (at black market prices), was now in to hoarding generic chocolate chip cookies. Interesting that she didn't eat them that much; she just wanted to *have* them—and in her own private place.

Age, infirmity, and decreasing autonomy do not eliminate the basic need for a place to keep secrets. Most personal papers and possessions gradually pass through the domain of caregiver, executor of the estate and, ultimately, beneficiaries; but never, while consciousness remains, should the patient be without a private place to maintain and manage at least a few personal effects. And such items are not always the most important or valuable, from an objective point of view, as we learned from Mother. Jewelry, china, and medical records were well enough dealt with by someone else, but heaven help the one who came between Mother and her stolen goodies.

As usual, there's the flip side of the issue. Privacy is one thing; too much (or unwanted) privacy is another. After Mother passed away, we converted her bedroom into a television and sitting room for Dad. With Dad's favorite reclining chair next to the open door, we tried to reduce his exposure to the parade of family down the hall and adjoining family room by placing a lamp and large plant to the right of his chair. Alas, sociable Dad didn't want to be obscured, protected, or otherwise kept out of the action. The day after we painstakingly arranged his new room, we found that he had moved the lamp and jungle-like plant to the *left* of his chair, all the better to wave and smile at—and keep an eye on—the nonstop human procession. (Somewhat ruefully, my husband and I later confided to each other that we had not only wanted to give Dad some relief but had hoped to buy a little privacy for *ourselves* in the original arrangement. We decided that we'd rather have him feel comfortable, at home, and a part of things—if that's what he wanted—than enjoy the occasional luxury of snacking in our underwear. We have plenty of time for that now.)

In the words of another...

I cannot feel like a prisoner in my own home. Our home must continue to be our refuge, even if an elderly parent is sharing it. This means, for example, that we do not have to change our way of doing everything—like deciding which news broadcast to watch, how to load the dishwasher, and so on. Also, I would not ban grandchildren from the house—even if they're noisy—but the elderly person's room could be made off-limits and as quiet as possible.

Another problem we had to deal with was a parent who hoarded, hid, and randomly destroyed objects (sometimes articles and documents of real value). Nothing was safe. We were about to put locks everywhere, but then I really would have felt like a prisoner. Thankfully, it did not come to that.

Marj

Additional Suggestion:

- A simple idea, but one you may overlook in the myriad of detail that comes with deciding which room(s) in your home to share with a loved one: Consider such things as traffic flow, the noise factor (where do children play?), access to a bathroom, and the like. If you are so fortunate as to already have a guest room, is that the wisest choice for an incapacitated guest arriving for a stay of unknown duration?

Your Ideas:

-

-

-

Lessons on Forgiveness

It was the lowest of all low blows. Perhaps I had neglected my own health—grabbed snacks on the run, usually in a walking sleep—while caring for my parents. And just maybe I was paying for that practice in fatigue and greater girth. But when Mother informed me on one of her last days that I appeared to be gaining weight, her comment seemed more a reprimand than a neutral observation. It was as if I had consciously pursued such an unsavory course in order to shame the family, and Mother was making it clear that this was not acceptable.

Then there was the time my Father—my sweet, uncomplaining, ever-complimentary Father—snapped at me and accused me of some reprehensible deed as I tried to make him more comfortable in his bed. I can't remember exactly what he said, and it really doesn't matter; all I know is that his words stung me to tears. It was so unlike him!

While these scenarios did not repeat themselves often during the years I cared for my parents, they occurred frequently enough toward the end that I began to look for an explanation. And I found it, at least in part. Did it come from a television documentary on geriatric care? a magazine article? advice from a friend who had passed through the same narrow and turbulent channel? Probably all of the above at one point or another.

Here's what I learned: The dearest people in the world—if they become sick or crippled enough, or spend one too many days in confinement—start to grow a weird emotional limb. They can experience intense frustration, fear, and possibly even feelings of worthlessness. Exacerbating the situation, medications and other treatments tend to compromise mental and social equilibrium. Frightening dreams often viewed in snatches punctuate restless nights, and dawns and twilights may become an endless now. Small wonder sweet folk we know and love start to exhibit uncharacteristically unflattering traits, and sometimes at our expense.[7]

Another memorable case in point: None of us present on that fateful Christmas Eve—Mother's last—will forget the long-awaited visit from our neighbor, Mrs. Champion. Predictably, she arrived at the door with her annual gift, a tin of holiday spiced walnuts. Dad, as I recall, was in the middle of his annual offering—reading the Christmas story aloud from the book of Luke—when the fragrant morsels began making their rounds among the eager assembly. Alas, the festive circulation was aborted as Mother lunged for, seized, and clutched the tin possessively to her floral muu muu, glaring as if to dare anyone to challenge her latest acquisition. Without so much as a discreet murmur of objection from any of us, Mother fished for and noisily consumed virtually every sugary nut to the ongoing recitation of gold, frankincense, myrrh—and other gifts of the season.

The prescription for childishness and offensive behavior? Regular doses of love. Comfort by the bucketful. Frequent reassurances that the cared-for one is secure and will not be abandoned. Atypical and undesirable behavior, I've come to believe, may indicate a test of commitment. When Mother began to wax selfish or abusive, for instance, she may have been daring us to leave her. Who knows? In any case, we never did—not for long, anyway—and I hope she found some measure of peace in our unconditional care and acceptance.

"Yes, Mother, I've gained weight. Stress can be fattening. And I love you anyway."

---

[7] Important to note here is that those who exhibit signs of mental or emotional distress—those with Alzheimer's, for instance—may be *incapable* of responding with improved behavior to your love and patience. And that's okay; maintain *your* level-headed compassion, and you'll both feel better.

Additional Suggestion:

• Be aware that certain negative effects—beyond feelings of frustration, anger, and guilt—can remain in your life long after your loved one has passed on. Jenny, a friend with whom I shared details of my experience, mentioned that her mother continues to be influenced by what *her* mother would have done in this situation or that—in spite of the fact that her mother (Jenny's grandmother) died years ago. While parental influence is inherently not a bad thing (it can be wonderful, in fact), too much *posthumous* influence can limit independent judgment, result in missed opportunities, and otherwise prove less than constructive.

Your Ideas:

•

•

•

A Case for Scheduling

"Remember, your bath is in five minutes. And Carol is still planning to read your life story to you at 4:30."

Weekly, daily, hourly, a schedule is your lifeline to organization and sanity—and a source of security and comfort to your patient. With incapacity can come feelings of despair, helplessness, and frustration, frequently accompanied by predicable "secondary" effects, including unpleasant and demanding behavior. When the cared-for one can plan on regular, sufficient care, negative emotions and actions are replaced with greater security and cooperation. You both win.

Try to get by without a schedule, on the other hand, and not only will your loved one suffer, you yourself will also soon learn firsthand the meaning of "beck and call." Before I implemented a routine, I simply responded to every request on demand; wasn't this, after all, the most loving and dutiful way to serve one's parents? That was in my "novice" days and, had it continued much longer, I would have preceded my parents in moving beyond this mortal sphere. I recall with a shiver one day in particular. I was driving, exhausted and in near delirium, from errand to errand in what I perceived to be the benevolent cause of stimulus-response. While waiting for the traffic light to change at the intersection of Broadway and Civic—I remember it well—I mused: "Well, if I wear myself out and just drop dead one of these days, at least no one can ask more of me." When this thought penetrated my consciousness, I realized it was time to change my approach to caring for the parents I loved.

My advice: Take a sheet of paper and write it all down—what needs to happen for your loved one every day, every week. Don't worry at first about the "whens"; just jot down the essentials, followed by the "nice-if-we-can-do-it" items. Next, identify services that must occur at certain times, e.g., meals if your patient is diabetic or otherwise in need of regular nourishment. Arrange more flexible needs around the fixed areas, and include a list of accessory services. I found it helpful to use a monthly calendar as well as a daily/weekly plan sheet to note irregular but important items, such as doctor appointments, occasional senior socials, or church activities my father enjoyed, and the like.

Following, then, are a few elements of our daily schedule—many of them simple ideas, to be sure, but so important to Mother and Dad (and to the rest of us, for reasons that will become clear). No doubt you'll add to the list as you develop your expertise.

- *The daily bath*—a much-anticipated ritual, and not just for the purpose of getting clean. Until the end when physical assistance was required, Dad was able to attend to his bath or shower with minimal assistance (from my husband, in most cases). "Aaaah," came the satisfied sigh, his moist brow aglow as he would exit the steamy bathroom in his burgundy robe. "There's nothing like it!"

Suggestions

Schedule the bath or shower—daily, if possible—when the patient is relaxed, and the caregiver has time to attend to necessary helping functions (ranging from full to only minor support). First thing in the morning is usually a good time. Provide clean clothes after the bath and, if possible, fresh (or at least "fluffed") bed linens. When assistance begins to require lifting the patient (or providing more in-depth care for a loved one of the opposite sex), the time has come to find more help—another relative or a paid attendant, perhaps. More on that later. One of the best ideas I discovered for helping Mother at bathtime was the four-legged raised toilet seat which, when transferred from toilet to tub, did marvelous double duty. Actually, only the rear legs of the chair fit into the bathtub, but Mother was able to sit on the seat, her legs extended outside the tub, while we washed the rest of her body with warm running water. It was quite a pleasant contrast—for both of us—to sponge baths in bed!

- *Mealtimes*—another favorite for most patients, who welcome not only the comfort of food, but a break in monotony and, ideally, an opportunity to socialize if only briefly with at least part of the family.

Suggestions

Establish an eating schedule around which other activities (e.g., exercise, napping, taking medications) are arranged. Ensure that only wholesome, nourishing foods are prepared for and served to your patient, taking care to follow any special instructions the patient's physician may indicate. Invite your loved one to participate as much as possible in the selection and preparation of meals; ask her or him to share favorite recipes and menus. Try to eat together as often as possible or, if your loved one is confined to bed, assign family members to take turns bringing meals to him and remaining long enough to meet social as well as nutritional needs.

- *Exercise*—an essential component of everyone's life, even if one's capacity is limited to lifting her fingers five times. Dad and I used to walk, albeit slowly, around Civic Park a couple of times most mornings. What wouldn't have been much of an aerobic workout to most turned out to be "sport extraordinaire" to Dad. Breathing deeply and following the brisk tap-tap-tap of his sporty cane, Dad pursued the pansied path as if it were a racetrack.

- *Naptime*—often more for the sanity of the caregiver than the patient's welfare. If physical needs have been met and the patient doesn't want to sleep, insist that the established "quiet time" be observed nonetheless.

- *Medication*—a definite item to be included in the daily schedule, when inadvertent lapses can be a matter of life or death. A thoughtful friend made my multiple pill-dispensing job much easier when she presented me with a storage/dispenser unit that held a week's worth of tablets and capsules storable by the morning, afternoon, evening, and bedtime of each day. When your patient takes upwards of thirteen different pills, capsules, and tablets every twenty-four hours, this little organizer can be a lifesaver for you both.

- *Entertainment*—good humor, company—if only for a few minutes each day. Let your loved one know that you—or someone—will be there to share conversation, stories of "auld lang syne," or simply a good joke. More than just a nice idea, offering companionship and humor can actually afford therapeutic benefits. Quoting again a favorite proverb, "A merry heart doeth good like medicine..." (Prov. 17:22).

Suggestions

Find a video or television program your loved one enjoys to supplement human companionship and entertainment. My mother, for instance, loved to watch the movie, *Maytime,* an old favorite starring Jeanette McDonald and Nelson Eddy. During the two hours and sixteen minutes the video ran each day, I could count on Jeanette and Nelson to keep Mother happily consumed, and I was able to attend to such personal luxuries as sweeping floors, cleaning bathrooms, and getting a start on the next creative, low-fat casserole, designed to sustain the four generations living in our household.

For variety, consider helping your loved one write or dictate her life story—and then read it back to her each day. This helps keep memory alert and allows the loved one to take pride in past accomplishments. A bonus: Those who read the autobiographical accounts—children or grandchildren, in most cases— are frequently amused, amazed, impressed, and delighted by the experiences and achievements of their forebear's life, the details of which perhaps had gone undiscovered to that point.

Your Ideas:

-
-
-

Looking Good, Feeling Better

This is probably the place to remind you that, as I noted in the introduction, this book was not intended to include comprehensive instructions on handling your loved one's physical and medical concerns. Numerous books, articles, community courses, and other resources can instruct on the mechanics of home health care. I have chosen to refer you to some of these (see Suggested Readings and Resources) rather than duplicate what already exists.

What I can offer within these pages are a few simple ideas I've found—some so basic as to be easily overlooked—generated via trial and error during the years I cared for my parents. The preceding chapter begins the process, suggesting ways to manage the timing of meals, exercise, rest, and medication. I'll touch on a related area in this chapter: helping your loved one look as attractive as possible. I used to think that feeling well preceded looking good, but now I'm convinced that the relationship is reciprocal. I'd say, in fact, that a clean and pleasing exterior actually promotes greater health and well-being. As caregiver, nurturer, daughter or son, do what you reasonably can to encourage your loved one to take pride in his or her appearance.

We were only going down the street to see her doctor, but Mother was dressed to the nines. Now, your mother may be a bit more practical and have a better sense of what's appropriate to wear where. But to mine, leaving the house was an event to be celebrated by donning her flaming red coat (whenever the temperature "dipped" below 85 degrees) and flamboyant purple scarf. Not to mention the exotic, cream-colored turban that inevitably completed the ensemble.

The important thing was, Mother *felt* better when she dressed up. And that was good, to a point; when Mother was feeling charming, though, she could flirt outrageously with whomever—the doctor, neighbor, furnace repairman. It got a little embarrassing.

Even at home in her bedroom, she experimented with this robe or that, and insisted on donning her zip-up-the-front Alice-blue caftan and ivory cameo when friends or family came to visit. And then we'd see the snap-on front tooth, the glossy dippity-do wave next to the side part, the mists of Heaven Sent settling on her glorious persona.

Once a fox, always a fox.

Additional Suggestions:

- Help your loved one feel especially well-groomed at least once a day—preferably in the morning. Find out what he or she needs in order to feel presentable and attractive, and do all you can to provide the necessary resources.

- Create a simple grooming kit to place by the patient's chair or bedside. A small pail or box might be used to hold such necessities as comb or brush, toothpicks or floss, cologne, wet wipes, tissue, breath mints, mirror, and the like.

- Encourage a neat immediate environment (within the sanitary and well-organized larger scene). Provide adequate shelving and closet space, and convenient trash disposal. Respectfully require your loved one to maintain a clean and orderly space to the extent that she or he is able.

Small Comforts and Celebrations

His body grew weak, but Dad's wanderlust continued to flourish until he conceded that he was decidedly, irreversibly, confined to home. Like the day some years earlier he had announced that, in the interest of public safety, he would finally surrender his driver's license, he knew when the time had come to cash in his traveler's checks and frame his passport.

Until then, though, my brothers and I took turns accompanying Dad on sentimental journeys. Granted, travel is generally not high on the list of activities pursued by the physically or mentally declining. And I seriously considered not mentioning in this book the fact that Armand, Gordon, and I alternated traveling with Dad to such places as Japan, where he had served as a missionary and later, mission president; Germany, a land rich in personal ancestral significance; and, ultimately, the Holy Land so that Dad, a devout Christian, could "walk where Jesus walked." Uncommon as this scenario may be in the typical caring environment, however, opportunities to help your loved ones truly live—albeit in unconventional ways, occasionally—can and do occur. Finances and health may not allow many ninety-year-old cancer patients to globe-trot, but Dad had planned ahead to enjoy his old age. He had contributed generously to his family and his savings account; and when he was able, finally, to embark on the trips of his dreams, we supported his desire as far as we were able.

One thing we learned early on in the travel-with-Dad scene was that the actual business of traveling, including arrival at the destination, usually wasn't as significant to Dad as the anticipation and preparation. Barring radiation or some other treatment that required Dad to remain at home, we typically made plans to go somewhere, near or far, every few months or so. Looking forward to going literally kept him going. Other loved ones, yours and mine, may not need to anticipate adventure beyond the local art museum or ice-cream parlor every three months to find the needed dose of recreation.

Less dramatic and costly activities added zest and longevity to my parents' lives as well. We found a reason to celebrate something almost every day. The arrival of May, for instance, was marked by a bowl of freshly cut camellias on the breakfast table; a therapeutic walk around the block yielded an extra-long foot rub at bedtime.

Then there were birthdays. Mother's featured the usual fanfare—a special dinner at home or, occasionally, at a favorite restaurant with as many loved ones in attendance as possible; a decorative cake, frequently prepared by a would-be artistic grandchild; and a few brightly wrapped gifts—a brushed flannel nightgown, a fragrant box of dusting powder (Heaven Sent, of course), perhaps a sweet treat or two from the local confectionery.

Dad's birthday, on the other hand, was a major event, and in his later years, a media event as well, especially when his new age ended in a five or a zero. Dad and two of his sisters, born October 16, 1900, were the first surviving triplets born in the state of Utah. From their childhood debut at the Utah State Fair until their ninetieth birthday celebration in Salt Lake City, the threesome shared a fast wit that made them a favorite with the local and national press. Perhaps the most memorable birthday was their eighty-fifth, on which the trio were featured on ABC-TV's "Good Morning, America" and in a two-page spread in *People* magazine.

Publicity and fanfare were fun, but we didn't need the world's attention to help Dad feel cared for and loved. I think the frequent smaller delights—that extra cherry on his tapioca to observe the arrival of *sakura* (cherry blossom) time—did the job just fine.

Additional Suggestions:

- Ensure that scrapbooks, photo albums, journals, and other personal and family history items are available to your loved one for frequent perusal.

- For a birthday or other special occasion, invite immediate and extended members of the family to each create a page for an *I Love You Because...* book. Encourage creativity and careful preparation. Bind contributions in scrapbook form, include a decorative cover, and watch the recipient enjoy paging through this loving tribute again and again.

- Help create or supplement a biographical record of the loved one. "Interview" him or her on audio- or videotape (preferably the latter), not only for the benefit of posterity, but for the subject's repeated enjoyment.

- Encourage your loved one's friends and relatives to drop by during "visiting hours"—times other than those scheduled for meals, exercise, rest, physical therapy, and the like. Be sure that your patient actually wants to entertain guests (some are more welcome than others!), and do not allow friends to overstay a reasonable visiting time or otherwise tire the patient. If the visit calls for privacy, ensure that interruptions are kept to a minimum and that both the visitor and visited are able to converse undisturbed.

- Develop soothing daily and weekly rituals—the cup of warm herbal tea with the evening news, a brief shoulder rub after bathing, a favorite weekly periodical delivered each Monday at breakfast. These and similar comforts incorporated into the routine add stability, anticipation, and color to an often otherwise neutral palette.

- Play favorite music in the background during bathtime, preparation for sleep, and at any other point in the day so your loved one can enjoy familiar, inspiring, or stimulating sounds.

Your Ideas:

-

-

-

Caring from a Distance

As I see it, there are two kinds of long-distance care, when you consider "long distance" to be anything other than under your own roof. Supplemental, in-town assistance is one kind; out-of-town, or out-of-state or country, is the other. Here are some initial thoughts you may wish to consider. You'll find more specific help in some of the resources I have identified at the end of this book.[8]

When your loved one lives in town, or close enough to be accessible, and is still more or less independent, your caregiving assistance can be relatively low stress, especially when other relatives live nearby and are also willing to help. When my parents maintained their own address for the years that my husband and I lived in the same community, my every-other-day visits started out simply enough: How well were they eating? Did they need help with cleaning and laundry? What about medication—were they both getting what they needed on time? Gradually, the visits became of the daily and longer variety, and I found myself preparing three meals a day, doing all the laundry, dispensing medication, and otherwise becoming indispensable. For a while, we helped them arrange part-time outside assistance; a trusted aide[9] would come in for a few hours each day to take care of housekeeping essentials, leaving me free to attend to the more personal and nurturing details of their care. And that was fine, as long as it lasted. The time eventually came, however, when periodic outside help was no longer an option; they needed live-in care. That's when we

---

[8] Take a look, for example, at a wonderful little book entitled *Caring for Your Aging Parents* by Kerri S. Smith, and the booklet, *Miles Away and Still Caring*.

[9] See Part IV: When You Can't Do It All: Hiring an Attendant for more information on obtaining outside assistance.

decided to invite them to our home—a choice that may or may not be wise or even possible for you.[10]

Should you find yourself in this first category, the giver of in-town assistance, may I suggest the following:

- Assess needs carefully, involving the loved one as much as possible. Don't make the mistake of swooping in *a la* "Lady Bountiful" at the first hint of need, promising services you cannot possibly provide in the long term, and which your loved one may not even require at this point.

- When you have determined as best you can the kind and amount of assistance needed, consider the options: To what other resources and helps does the patient have potential access? How much help can you reasonably give? Can you realistically promise to provide the main meal five days a week and arrange a weekly housecleaning? One of the finest services you can render is to help your loved one list every possible source of assistance and encourage him or her to pursue a variety of options. You might also offer to help access those options, e.g., ask others to assist you in the caregiving process. If a parent needs meals prepared, for instance, and you have brothers and sisters in the area, you could offer to plan a meal preparation or delivery schedule with your siblings, and follow up to make sure that the schedule works. Or, you might introduce your parent to Meals on Wheels (or a similar program), and arrange to have the service begin. *Bottom line: Help your loved one retain as much dignity and self-reliance as possible by positioning yourself as a resource rather than a take-charge-of-the-victim superior.*

[10] Review Part I: Making the Caring Decision.

- When you have assessed your loved one's needs, considered options available, and established your role as facilitator, commit yourself to complete certain daily or weekly tasks. Consider your personal, family, and career obligations, and then communicate clearly to Mother, for instance, that you will visit her on Monday, Wednesday, and Friday from noon to 2 p.m., during which time you can style her hair, clean up the kitchen, and read from her favorite books. She can plan on you, and you can plan on removing a source of guilt and frustration from your life.

I can just hear my friend, Martina, saying something like this about now:

> *You must be kidding. My mother has just had her third stroke, the children are down with the flu, and my husband is in Hong Kong on business. I'm supposed to sit down and calmly, rationally, "assess" all my "options?" I'm kneeling here at midnight, mopping up the disgusting outcomes of Bobby's upset stomach, and wondering how I'm going to bring Mother home from the hospital on Friday—the day I simply have to do office payroll.*

I hear you, Martina. I spent most of my time responding, knee-jerk fashion, to crises as they occurred. I found myself changing bedsheets in the middle of the night when I was so weary I thought I wouldn't see the dawn; cooking six meals a day based on varying dietary restrictions and preferences; postponing carpal-tunnel surgery for my injured wrists so that I could continue to give foot rubs and back massages without interruption. *I hear you!* I know that some of my suggestions sound academic and out of touch with reality when you're thick in the middle of those terribly trying moments. When things get that bad—and they do, at times—you need more than guidelines to assist you. You need your wits, some well-developed survival skills, outside assistance (human and divine), and perhaps some adjusted expectations for yourself. A good night's sleep can make all the difference, too.

The second kind of long-distance care, the out-of-area variety, is a different story, indeed. Assuming your loved one simply needs some help from time to time, you might consider visiting him or her and creating a "help hotline," a notebook you can leave with the patient (taking a copy home with you for reference). In this resource, you might record outcomes of the following:

- A visit with the doctor(s), in which you identify yourself as the primary caregiver of the patient. State that you live out of town but wish to be involved in the patient's care. You might ask to leave your name, telephone number, and address with the patient's health care practitioners, along with a request that you be notified in the event of emergency or significant change in the patient's health.

- A visit to your loved one's neighbors, if appropriate—those he or she may know and not know very well. Ask if they would be willing to give their telephone numbers for the loved one to call in case of immediate need.

- A check of your loved one's home or apartment, in which you correct any obvious dangers (frayed electrical cords or ill-placed furniture, for example), and perhaps a note on the careful use of potentially hazardous equipment (a reminder to turn off the stove, if the loved one shows signs of forgetfulness).

- A written list of all medications the patient must take, and a schedule which clearly identifies when and with what the medication should or should not be taken.

- A suggested meal plan and easily rotated shopping list, if the patient is able to shop and cook for him- or herself.

When the loved one's condition deteriorates to the point that he or she cannot function any longer with such interim measures, everyone involved has a decision to make. One option you might consider, if the patient chooses to stay at home, is to recommend the use of a "geriatric case manager," a relatively new professional title bestowed on individuals willing to coordinate the care of homebound elderly. For a fee, the manager oversees the patient's physical, medical, and legal well-being, working closely with attendants, physicians, housecleaning services, attorneys, and the like, to ensure that needs are met. If you choose to procure the services of a geriatric case manager on behalf of a parent, for instance, you can expect to receive a periodic report on your parent's status and notification of any immediate need your parent might not be able to communicate without assistance.[11]

Your Ideas:

-

-

-

---

[11] See Suggested Readings and Resources for information available from the National Association of Geriatric Case Managers.

PART IV.
Sharing the Caring

For the sake of my own health and sanity, I simply cannot work both the nightshift and dayshift more often than very occasionally.
—Marj

Found: An Extra Two-and-a-half Hours a Day!

Now they tell me. *I* didn't have to do it all!

This is another one of those see-what-I-learned-after-the-fact chapters, which I begin with a plea derived from retrospect: Decide at the outset—*now, even before your caring challenge begins, perhaps*—to explore every conceivable source of assistance and support. Ultimately, you will have more to give as you appropriately share the burden and blessing of your undertaking. Subsequent chapters in this section describe more successful efforts I made to involve family, friends, and professionals in the care of my parents. I hope you will apply or modify these ideas in ways that will be of most use in your situation.

Meanwhile, this brief chapter concludes with a few "wish-I'd-dones." No doubt you'll be able to add some of your own to the list.

Ideas for you to consider:

- Contact a local college or high school to locate students who would be willing to run errands, visit, or read to your loved one, and otherwise assist you in the caregiving process. You may not need to look further than a neighbor teen or young adult to obtain this volunteer or for-hire assistance.

- Find out if your community has a respite-care program providing adult day care by social workers and other qualified professionals. Arts and crafts projects, simple

66

exercises, songfests, and other activities (as well as meals and snacks) are offered to participants, many of whom enjoy the diversion as much as the caregiver, who will thus find time to attend to personal affairs.[12]

- Find out if local senior centers offer the services of capable volunteers (many of whom, incidentally, are seniors themselves) to tend and entertain the aged or infirm. Contact your church or synagogue to determine the availability of similar programs.

- Your county health center can refer you to additional resources for seniors, including regular meal delivery, in-home personal services, low-cost recreation and transportation, and the like.

So I found out, mostly after the fact, that I could have had more help. Now you know better and, chances are, it isn't too late for you to take advantage of the resources at your disposal. Learn from my experience. Free up those extra hours—sometimes extra moments—and spend them somewhere else. On yourself, perhaps. Yes, that would be a good place to start.

---

[12] For more information, call the toll-free referral service offered by the National Council on the Aging, at 1-800-424-9046.

Baseball in the Park (and Other Kinds of Helpful Togetherness)

Why we didn't capture the scene on camera I'll never know. There was Dad on one of his better days, poised picture-perfect at the pitcher's mound, softball in hand. Next to him stood six-year-old Joseph, his great-grandson, straining to imitate every detail of stance, angle, and expression modeled by the once semipro baseball player. Each was completely absorbed in this moment of glory; neither mentor nor protege was aware of the curious glances and chuckles their performance elicited from passersby. It was a memory *du jour*—one repeated in some context or another nearly every day the two lived in our home.

The happy activities of Generations One and Four created more than fodder for precious reminiscences, however. When Dad and Joseph, or Dad and any one of the children, were busily involved, I was a free woman, "free" being a relative thing. I cherished the moments Dad and the grandchildren enjoyed at the ice-cream parlor because I knew how much they looked forward to this weekly event *and* because their absence created a welcome hour of alone time for me.

And they did more than entertain each other: Joseph and Angela helped button Dad's shirts when his palsied hands shook too much to do the job themselves. Dad frequently volunteered to comb or cut Joseph's hair, with unfortunate consequences for Joseph on the days Dad's palsy acted up. Little Mariana learned her ABCs perched upon Dad's stubby legs in front of his bulbous middle (he just missed having a lap). Each of the children enjoyed helping take meals into Dad's room when Dad was unable to join us at the family table. Heading the parade with the heaviest cargo—entree and salad on a tray—was Angela, with her superior coordination and strength. Joseph followed, usually managing to deliver most of the beverage still inside the glass. Mariana toddled behind, a supply of napkins in her diminutive fist and the satisfied smile of a job well done on her face as she deposited her contribution on target. "Oh boy, oh boy, oh boy," Dad always murmured appreciatively at the spread arranged before him. "Just call if you want summor of dis," Mariana would grin, taking a swipe of gravied mashed potatoes with a tiny finger. "Mmmm, dat's good, Granfathah!"

My grandchildren. Dad's *great*-grandchildren. An unlikely but such a rich source of assistance to both Dad and me. And the children are forever rewarded by tender memories of mutual service, story time, and those ball games in the park.

In the words of another…

> *Mother doesn't live with us—yet, anyway. We want her to maintain as much independence as possible for as long as her strength will permit, and she is more than happy at that thought. But living alone shouldn't mean being alone all the time. We involve her as much as we can in family events, like summer picnics, the children's school programs, church socials, and the like. So far, it has been a good arrangement; we've all had as much "togetherness" as we want and need.*
>
> *—MaryDee*

Additional Suggestions:

- If you're caring for a parent, involve your willing brothers and sisters in the care process as much as possible—even if they live out of the immediate area and need to make some sacrifices in time and travel. A personal nonexample: My older and younger brothers, both living hundreds of miles away, offered more help than I accepted. I reasoned that they had their own challenges and local obligations, and certainly couldn't be expected to do as much as I. Perhaps so but looking back, I see that this was a costly attitude, not only in terms of my own limited strength, but in what it essentially denied my brothers on a certain, then largely unrecognized, parent-child dimension. Given a second chance, I would have accepted their offers (or even enlisted a few more) to spend an occasional week caring for Mother and Dad. When we realized that we were dealing with a chronic, possibly very long-term situation, we could have arranged for each brother or his family to assist our parents for a week (or even a weekend) every third month or so. Again, my brothers were willing and as generous as I would let them be. I just wish I had taken time— then—to set aside whatever excessively unselfish or martyr-like motivations managed my unconscious and think.

In the words of another...

> *Dad isn't really sick right now, but he's ninety-six and unable to attend to some of his basic needs without help. So my four very busy brothers and I proposed this idea to him: Why not come stay with each of us for three to six months at a time? That way, you don't get bored since you get to spend time in virtually every corner of the country—and we can manage temporary changes in our schedules more easily when adjustments are occasional rather than permanent. We're into this arrangement a year and a half now and, I'm pleased to say, so far so good.*
>
> *—Lois*

- If full-time togetherness with a family member is not possible or desirable, consider the part-time option. Cheryl, a friend who works full-time in a demanding career and is single, finally realized after a near disaster that she could no longer accommodate her homebound Aunt Susie in the spare bedroom. Reluctantly, she helped Aunt Susie make alternative living arrangements in a local nursing home, which could provide regular opportunities for social interaction as well as a physically safe environment for one who might fall or accidentally overdose on medication if left alone. To help her aunt retain a sense of home and belonging, though, Cheryl brings Susie home whenever possible on weekends—when Cheryl can be there to supervise—and on holidays. When a weekend at home is not an option, Cheryl spends two or three hours on Saturday taking Susie shopping or to her favorite restaurant.

- In addition to offering physical and emotional support to the loved one in your care, family members may contribute financially, if such is called for. My parents were prepared for retirement and prolonged health care, but other situations may call for external assistance. Some adult children who care for a parent, for instance, each contribute an agreed-upon number of dollars per month toward the cost of the parent's maintenance.

Caveat: If your parent receives assistance from Medicaid, you no doubt are already aware that ongoing participation in the program restricts the amount of money he or she can collect from other sources. Of course, Medicaid and other sources of government support exist to assist those who have no other recourse, so compliance with program requirements—the participant can have no more than $2,000 in savings, for instance—is generally not a serious challenge. If, however, you begin to supplement the beneficiary's income, even sporadically, you may find the burden of continued support squarely upon *your* shoulders. Unless you are able to maintain this responsibility (in which case, the taxpayers of America thank you), ensure that you are thoroughly familiar with rules and regulations surrounding government assistance to your loved one before, rather than after, you find yourself in a more financially responsible position than you can maintain.

Your Ideas:

•

•

•

Dealing with Doctors: A Prescription

Perhaps your loved one enjoys the good fortune of a successful, long-established relationship with a competent physician. If so, that's a plus, especially when health begins to decline and the need for reliable care becomes critical. If, on the other hand, this relationship is lacking when the need arises—and you have assumed the task of helping to meet that need—you may find yourself in the position of shopping for medical care. Assuming you have already navigated this course for yourself (and for your children, perhaps), you probably have some good ideas on how to go about it on behalf of someone else. Still, you may find it helpful to review my ideas on how to establish a working doctor/patient/caregiver arrangement with a doctor who wants to help you and your loved one, who will cooperate with specialists and other health-care providers, and who can give your loved one the best care possible. Here are some suggestions:

- *Select (or help select) the primary-care physician carefully, if you can.* As most of us can attest, there are doctors, and then there are *doctors.* You'll want competence, first of all, and you can check for that by reviewing qualifications, seeking references, and getting a sense of his or her reputation. Next, I'd suggest you look for accessibility: Is the doctor available, within reason, when you need him or her? Then there's the matter of personality, or "bedside manner," which includes sensitivity, kindness, and a willingness to work with you and the patient. Find someone who scores high in all three categories, and you have a winner.

If your loved one belongs to a health maintenance organization (HMO) or is otherwise limited in the choice of physicians, you will both need to learn the art of managing yourselves within the system. Mother and Dad had been members of an HMO for years, which served them best usually in urgent care or emergency situations. Obtaining efficient *routine* care posed a greater challenge, since appointments often had to be made weeks in advance, and sheer patient volume necessarily diluted the personal touch.

- *Help your patient follow doctor's orders, and report outcomes to the doctor whether or not he or she asks for a follow-up.* An occasional note summarizing your patient's condition—or even a simple note of thanks—is also a nice idea, and a good way to be remembered. If your loved one is able to do the calling or writing, so much the better. I wish I'd backed off sometimes and let Dad do the talking.

- *Ask the doctor to identify likely side effects of prescribed medications.* Is this syrup expected to produce nausea? Should we be concerned if Dad becomes drowsy after taking these little red capsules? It is especially critical to anticipate possible side effects and the results of various drug interactions when you're working with someone like my father, a cancer/heart/lung/kidney patient, who required the services of more than one physician or course of treatment. "Doctor B," for example, prescribed the drug Interferon for Dad, unaware that "Doctor A" had Dad receiving regular radiation treatments. With both doctors out of town over a long holiday weekend, we could only speculate—correctly, it turned out—that this was a potentially lethal combination. Specialists often do their best to coordinate care, but we learned that the patient (and the patient's caregiver) are ultimately responsible to ensure that all health-care professionals involved have a clear understanding of medications and treatments prescribed, and are kept informed of the patient's response.[13]

Additional Suggestions:

- Keep the patient's medical records and all related information in an easily accessed folder or large envelope. Include his or her full name and social security number, names and telephone numbers of primary and specialized-care physicians, a brief and current medical history, current prescriptions and dosages, allergies, and so on. Take careful notes during every visit with doctors and other health-care practitioners, marking the date and outcomes of the encounter. Should your patient need to enter the hospital suddenly or require immediate medical attention, you will have necessary details and documents already assembled. Simply being prepared for such an eventuality will offer peace of mind to you and your loved one.

- Ask doctors for any helpful written or personal resources they may neglect to mention, e.g., medical supply sources, dietary guidelines, community assistance (including reputable adult day-care programs), and the like. Find out, also, if medical social workers are available to answer additional questions or offer support the doctor may be too busy to personally provide.

---

[13] Your pharmacist can help with this. Most pharmacies today are equipped with computers that will signal potentially dangerous interactions from prescribed medications.

- While we want to help our loved ones maintain as much independence as possible, it's important to encourage them to manage personal health-care matters only to the extent that they are able. If a patient suffers from Alzheimer's or any other form of mental impairment, for example, ensure that medications remain in your safe-keeping and exclusively under your control.

Your Ideas:

-

-

-

When You Can't Do It All: Hiring an Attendant

Bernice, Arturo, Mary. They may be just names to you, but to me they are no less than angels. They and a few others served as attendants to my parents during those difficult final months. My only regret is that I didn't pursue the "get some help" option after the first missed night's sleep. I struggled valiantly—and unnecessarily—to function both day and night until I simply could go no further.

So, when do you seriously explore finding an attendant, aide, or nurse for your loved one? I suggest the time for help has come when—

- you and your immediate family (or voluntary support system) can no longer handle the full care of your loved one without jeopardizing your own health or neglecting important personal affairs;

- extended family (including your brothers and sisters, in the case of caring for a parent) are unable to provide sufficient assistance; or

- community and other external resources (see the first chapter of part four) are no longer adequate for your needs.

Before you hire outside assistance, I recommend that you contact Medicare or Medicaid to investigate the possibility of obtaining licensed home health care free of charge or at a reduced rate. Skilled nursing and various therapeutic services may be available, depending on whether your patient meets certain eligibility requirements. Your patient's physician and insurance carrier will be able to provide further details on the availability of these options.

If your loved one qualifies for the Medicare or Medicaid option, or if another low-cost, legitimate, and reliable source of assistance becomes available, great. But you may be required to search for, screen, hire, and manage the services of a skilled nurse or attendant. Following are a few suggestions to help make that task a little easier.

- First, decide exactly what kind of help is needed, and how often. Does your loved one's condition require skilled assistance, e.g., a nurse who can administer shots and regulate other treatments, or are you simply looking for a companion who can assist with meals and baths? Do you need round-the-clock help, or would a four-hour shift every afternoon provide the relief you need to attend to other matters? Toward the end with Mother and Dad, my husband and I found that our greatest need was a good night's sleep, so we hired an attendant to assist from 10 p.m. to 6 a.m., providing whatever care was needed during those hours. What a difference those eight hours of rest and freedom made!

- If you find that you need skilled nursing assistance, part or full time, you might start the search by asking your patient's physician or nurse for a recommendation. The nursing department of a local college or university could also provide you with ideas—including, perhaps, referral to nursing students looking for part-time employment. In addition, you may want to check your telephone directory for the Visiting Nurses Association which provides skilled nursing services to Medicare and Medicaid patients (and will also accept payment from medical insurance and private resources).

- Finding a less-skilled aide or attendant can be a little trickier. Some private nurses have been certified, but licensing is not required of all (or even most) attendants. Possibly the safest—and definitely the most expensive—course here is to contact a home health-care agency. The agency hires, screens, and pays its employees (most of whom are bonded), and you pay the agency directly. If you decide to forego agency fees and hire an attendant directly, proceed with caution. Note these caveats:

  - Seek referrals from trusted sources—ideally, a friend or acquaintance who successfully employs, or has employed, an individual for the same purpose. You could also check a local senior center where, in some cases, healthy "younger seniors" who want part-time work will advertise their services.

  - *Do not* advertise for help in the newspaper or respond to ads you see in the newspaper. While many such candidates are quite legitimate, more than one unscrupulous would-be attendant could appear on your doorstep long enough to abscond with your valuables or, perhaps, have an unfortunate "accident" on your premises that could add expensive and exasperating litigation to your list of challenges. Don't take the chance.

  - From whatever source you find a candidate for the position, *ask for and check* references before promising employment.

  - During the initial interview with the prospective attendant, include an introduction to your loved one. Does the applicant appear to take a genuine interest in him or her? How well does the applicant discuss his or her qualifications, requirements, expectations? Does his or her background and personality mesh well with your patient's needs? If the first meeting bodes well, invite the candidate to a second interview. Inform him or her that the next meeting will be an "audition" of sorts, for which you will pay an agreed-upon fee for an hour's work. During the second meeting, invite the applicant to complete a task or two that would likely be a typical part of a shift's work, e.g., cleaning and straightening the patient's room or preparing and serving a light meal. I found that this simple exercise reveals volumes about a candidate's skill, personality, and bedside manner, and cannot be duplicated during a verbal interview alone.

- If both interviews and the candidate's referrals prompt you to offer the position, ask the applicant for proof of U.S. citizenship or, in the case of an alien applicant, a green card. Call your state and federal tax office to arrange legal (taxed) compensation.

- You may want to offer employment on a trial basis at first, allowing you, the patient, and the attendant to explore working conditions and personalities with no obligation for the first week or two. Should you mutually decide to continue the arrangement after the trial period, agree upon an acceptable length of notice the attendant or you will give the other when termination becomes necessary.

- Continue to clarify expectations with the attendant as your relationship proceeds. Never assume that he or she will do exactly what you would do in a given situation; provide a written job description and patient schedule, and make explicit any additional duties that may arise. Encourage the attendant to share with you any difficulties or frustrations the job may create, and do whatever you can within reason to maintain the attendant's satisfaction. Truly, good help is hard to find—and worth keeping.

Additional Suggestions:

- Have the attendant keep a written record of services performed during his or her shift. Subsequent helpers (including yourself) will find it useful to know what the patient has eaten, how long he or she has slept, and what medications were taken in the preceding hours. Any abnormalities or difficulties should also be noted on the record. I recommend keeping the record in a three-ring binder stocked with plenty of paper to encourage caregivers to include copious narrative along with the more standard content, e.g., patient intake and output, body temperature, blood pressure, and the like.

- Remember, if Medicaid services are used, you and your patient must become thoroughly familiar with its policies and requirements for continued assistance.

Your Ideas:

-

-

-

Hospice: A Merciful Intervention

You may struggle for weeks, months, *years,* hoping and believing that the crisis will pass and your loved one will be restored to health. When things are finally "back to normal," you'll finally take that deep breath and continue living yourself.

And then one day you realize that recovery is simply not going to happen. Perhaps a physician presents you with the irrefutable facts: your loved one has only weeks to live, assuming all goes well. Or, after one too many trips to the emergency room, one close call right on the heels of another, you realize that death is not only inevitable, it may be imminent. Often, no one has to tell you; you just know. More often than not, the patient knows it, too. Strangely, though, an acceptance of this unbidden reality often brings its own unexpected comfort to you both. Is it the relief of battle ended? making peace with nature? an awareness that suffering is about to end and the loved one can finally anticipate some welcome rest?

Whatever your thoughts and reactions at this moment of truth, one thing is certain: another decision waits to be made. Unless your loved one is so desperately ill that hospitalization is absolutely required (and this is seldom the case), you generally have three options:

(1) You can choose to maintain the status quo at home—continuing to care for the patient as you have been to this point, only with more frequent trips to the emergency room and overall greater stress to everyone concerned.

(2) You may, at this point, place your loved one in the care of an institution (including, in some cases, a regular hospital) for round-the-clock monitoring.

(3) With the physician's authorization, you can keep the loved one at home and supplement current care efforts with

the services of a hospice program. Hospice allows the terminally ill to experience the process of dying, peacefully surrounded by family and friends at home (or in a simulated home environment), and removed from sterile and noisy hospitals or other more public-care facilities. The emphasis is on comfort-based care versus unrealistic and painful efforts to overcome disease and maintain life at any cost. Bringing the fundamentals of medical care to the home, Hospice offers emotional and practical support to patients and their families, encouraging patients to be as alert, pain-free, and comfortable as possible until the end.

Let me say right here, in case I haven't made my position sufficiently obvious, that I am prejudiced in favor of Hospice. We weren't aware of the program during Mother's last days, but Hospice truly saved the day when Dad was dying, providing just enough additional support to keep him at home *and* maintain my rapidly diminishing sanity. We could legitimately have put Dad in the hospital during his final weeks, but it was during that time, especially, that I wanted him to feel the uninterrupted flow of love and support from family and friends. I wanted him to eat and sleep and bathe according to the schedule to which he had become accustomed, not at the convenience of the hospital staff. I wanted him home.

A hospice program typically takes a team approach, consisting of doctors, nurses, social workers, bereavement counselors, therapists, and volunteers. In addition to the twenty-four-hour availability of treatment and counseling services provided by the team, Hospice benefits include access to medication, medical supplies, and medical equipment. I was amazed at the variety of truly helpful physical supports and comforts introduced to us by our Hospice representatives. When, for example, our hospice nurse noted that Dad was perilously close to contracting a full-blown (and very painful) case of bedsores, we received an electrically charged mattress pad for his bed. Its mild electrical currents gently massaged Dad's bruised limbs and brought him significant relief.

Does your loved one qualify for Hospice care? A life expectancy of six months or less is the general requirement for acceptance into a hospice program. Consult with your patient's physician regarding the timing and appropriateness of your loved one's entry into hospice care. If, after weighing the alternatives, you and your loved one decide that dying at home is the preferred choice, communicate this decision to the doctor and request referral to a reputable hospice program.

That's what we did, and we've had no regrets.[14]

---

[14] See Suggested Readings and Resources for the address and the telephone number of the National Hospice Organization.

PART V:
Parting Thoughts

We often enter one of life's challenges "without a clue," as the saying goes. Oh, we may think we know what we're getting into. Or we jump off our respective cliffs (with parachutes of varying integrity) under the impression that we'll somehow hit land on the run, stumble toward our destination, and then move on with life as we knew it.

Ah, but there's the rub: "Life as we knew it" becomes a thing of the past. Life is never quite the same, and that can be for the good. In my case, even perceived costs, on balance, have been worth it for the most part. So where am I now, compared to where I used to be? More patient and understanding (virtues I thought I had plenty of before), less controlling, and much more peaceful. Life is good; better, in many respects, than it has ever been.

Descent from the Good Housekeeping Pedestal

I had always considered myself a kind, understanding person, but I simply had no patience for those who might be characterized as—may I put it bluntly?—*slobs*. I took an almost righteous pride in maintaining a clean, well-run home and decent personal appearance, going so far, incidentally, as to preserve many a salon coiffure by wrapping my head in toilet paper before retiring for the night. And until the four-generation carnival came to town (and set up its tents, so to speak, in our living room), these virtues had never truly been put to the test.

What follows is the recounting of an incident that still makes me cringe—but just a little, now. It was, at that time, the *coup de grace* and the ultimate horror. In retrospect, I think it represents a turning point in my attitudes and expectations.

So there I stood at the front door greeting the Channel 7 news crew, toilet brush in hand, my hair in curlers. The nice man at the television station had assured me earlier on the phone that they wouldn't be arriving for some hours hence. He lied.[15]

This was the day that everyone in the San Francisco Bay Area who tuned in to the local ABC television affiliate for News at Six and Ten, would share in the celebration of the Mauss Triplets' ninetieth birthday celebration. Besides the fact that the crew's early arrival rendered me less than presentable, the star of the show—my father—was still working at the office; he wasn't even home! "No problem," cooed the well-mani-

---

[15] Let's give him the benefit of the doubt, instead; we'll just say he was confused. Or was I the one who got it all wrong?

cured director, eyeing me pitifully. "We'll just interview you for the time being, if we may…perhaps take some pictures of Mr. Mauss's family and surroundings, and what have you…."

"What have we," I thought to myself, my mind racing, "is a cluttered living room and two dirty bathrooms. But keep your grip," I told myself, clutching the toilet brush more tightly. "We also have wit, charm, a touch of *savoir-faire*—yes, and the Hall of Fame! Saved," I breathed gratefully to myself, "by Dad's memento collection and photo gallery!"

"You probably don't want to interview me in this condition," I smiled hopefully (and with greater confidence, I thought, than warranted by my appearance at the moment). "But I'll be happy to show you a special room you'd probably find quite interesting. Please, come with me right down the hall here. Watch your step; you don't want to damage that nice tripod bumping into the….Whoops! Are you okay?"

That day really happened. And, yes, I appeared on the news that evening, in all my Cinderella glory. It was not unlike many others I survived during the years that two, then four, generations lived under our roof simultaneously. I, who once had prided myself on maintaining a clean and orderly environment—to say nothing of appearance—was forced by circumstance to relax my standards a bit (actually, a lot) and just "roll with it." While I can't say I ever reached the point of being able to enjoy clutter and disarray, I did learn to tolerate it, especially when I kept my sights on the bigger picture and realized that all of this was only temporary. Interesting that now, unlike years past, I don't silently note and criticize those dust bunnies and spider webs and unwashed dishes I see in other homes. Or think, "Gee, if they could just get out of bed five minutes earlier, they wouldn't have to live like that…."

Tolerance, empathy, patience: virtues refined in extremity,

resulting in a kinder, gentler attitude toward myself and others. No longer do I consider a chronic bathtub ring—yours or mine—a moral infraction or reflection of character.

Letting Go: When the End Comes

How do you put a Band-Aid on a stroke?

—*Mary Ellen*

As humans, we're programmed to preserve, store, retain. When I was a young mother, my life revolved around the care and maintenance of teeth, strong bones, play clothes, and the like. As my children grew older, I patched fewer skinned knees and more skinned hearts. And when I became primary caregiver for my parents, my preservation instincts kicked into high gear. Here were those who had given me life, now needing my help to retain theirs. Could there be any who were more deserving of my efforts to help maintain health and well-being?

So I found it difficult—for at least those two reasons—to detach and adopt a cool, objective response to my parents' deterioration and approaching death. In a cognitive sense, I knew, in spite of my best efforts, that I couldn't keep them living indefinitely. I suppose I knew, too, that *they* didn't want to hang on forever, no matter what. But on another level, my "heartbound" one, perhaps, I wanted to help them feel as healthy, content, and—dare I confess it?—immortal as possible. I wasn't sure, in my less rational moments, how I would handle their departure, not only from the world, but from my care.

And so it was that for the first few months following the death of Mother and then Father, I plagued myself with thoughts like, "If I'd only had the doctor check for *this*, Mother might have avoided *that*," and "Couldn't we have done *something* to make Dad more comfortable that last week?" and "Why did I leave his side that night? I was so tired and couldn't have sat up one more minute, but why did I choose *that* night to go to bed?"

89

Then I discovered, after a period of painful self-recriminations, that the "if onlys" were slowly evaporating, to be replaced by more frequent reflections on happy memories. I laughed more, thinking about those ridiculous and tender moments, like when Mother said "artichokes" or "caterpillars" when referring to her hair curlers after the first stroke left her speech less organized. And Dad with that little green shamrock pin he liked to wear, even when it wasn't St. Patrick's Day. To this day, I can't drive past Civic Park without smiling as I recall the "laps" Dad and I used to hobble around the park perimeter. We started our jaunts, ostensibly for Dad, shortly after my knee surgery; the assistance I supposedly rendered Dad during his walking therapy would have been impossible had I not been able to lean on *him!*

How strange. And how wonderful that residual despair and regret have melted into a quiet pool of peaceful reflection.

Life (a Few Years) After Death

In the words of a friend who lost her mother shortly after they finally made peace following a lifetime of struggle…

> *After Christmas, Mother went downhill quickly. Once, she came out of her coma after I had just showered. I knelt beside her bed with my hair still wet; she gently fluffed my naturally curly hair, which she had always loved. For a brief moment, she was mellow, without pain. Then she slipped back into a coma, and soon she was gone.*
>
> *The most difficult part of my grief was the profound regret that Mother and I hadn't had much time to enjoy the healing fruits of our mutual forgiveness. The bridge we built just before her death could never be completely crossed in this lifetime. There would be no more tender times in the drugstore, watching her fill her cart with treasures, no more shared hamburgers at the soda fountain. I would never see her dance again.*
>
> —Vivian

My response to a parent's death: a three-month case of pneumonia, followed by mononucleosis. When Dad passed away, four years after Mother's departure, I suppose I simply shut down, too. For fourteen years, I had willingly accepted the semisweet burden of their care; but for sixty-one, I had tried to follow their parental example. On some level, perhaps, I felt it my daughterly duty to "call it a day"—call it a *life*, perhaps—when they did. Either that, or I was simply so spent in every way, I finally gave in to the rest my body had unsuccessfully demanded for years.

I'm pleased to report that I eventually recovered; my health and mental equilibrium have returned. My home life now, sans Generations One, Two,[16] and Four, consists of my husband and me, along with our silent and relatively nondemanding

---

[16] My daughter and her family have since moved to Utah.

peach and lemon trees. We still rise fairly early most mornings (if we feel like it), enjoy a leisurely bowl of oatmeal, and study the scriptures together for a few moments before I adjourn to the stationary bicycle.[17] Then it's on to business or social pursuits, or preparations for voluntary church service assignments.

It isn't always so idyllic and stress-free, but I must say, life has never been calmer, more peaceful, or more truly enjoyable for us. We frequently reflect on the challenging years behind us, pleased, for the most, with our response. We keep close by a variety of visual reminders of those we love; mementos from Dad's "hall of fame" have largely been distributed among posterity, but remaining items decorate our walls and hearth. A portrait of my mother in her prime adorns my bedroom wall. My friend, Vivian, has taken a different, more dramatic, approach to preserving her mother's memory. As she tells it,

> *The closest I could get to Mom [after her death] was through the few personal belongings I had inherited—a patchwork quilt, Jenny Lind bed, china cabinet, some linens saved for company, a few knick-knacks.... Using the colors of the patchwork quilt for our inspiration, my husband and I painted and papered our guest room, and then gathered together my mother's treasures to display in the china cabinet. I put the final touches on the room by placing her baby picture on the shelf beside the bed, and filling the room with flowers—the kind that brought her such delight.*
>
> *This memorial to her has become a sanctuary for me, a place to go for healing and peace. When I need my mother, I crawl between the covers and imagine her presence nearby. With time and divine intervention, my image of her sadness has been replaced by a new sense of serenity and joy. I dream of her spirit unshackled, dancing in divine meadows. At last, she is at peace—and so am I.*

---

[17] Still the faithful friend that helps me maintain my strength, flexibility, and feeling of well-being.

I conclude with this sobering observation: Now that my parents have taken their places among the angels, I lack that buffer I had once enjoyed between me and eternity. I am the generation "up at bat" with the life beyond, and believe me, it's a new sensation. What have I learned from my caregiving experience to help me live the final chapter with grace and providence? Let me share the insights of two other caregiving friends, both of whom brought to my attention essentially the same idea:

Said Marj,

> *Sometimes I wonder how I will be in my dotage. It seems clear that I will be "more"—but more what? There will be more of what went on before, for good and ill. The declining years on earth seem to be a time to reap as we have sown, both good and bad. I think of my aunt, a world-class hoverer, being hovered over, smotheringly and devotedly by her daughters as she had surely done for them, to the detriment of all concerned.*

Phyllis agreed, commenting,

> *I have observed that our dominant traits, whatever they may be, are magnified as we age and move toward the end of our lives. An impatient style, for example, becomes more pronounced, and can deteriorate into demanding senility. At a luncheon with some close friends not long ago, I noticed that the discussion turned to the subject of aging and caring for the aging—things that most, if not all, of us will do eventually. One of our number commented thoughtfully, "Are we listening? What will we be like when we reach the point of needing care?"*

Let me not forget.

Author's Note

Hello, I'm Susan. I crafted most of the wording in this book, but the experiences and suggestions herein originate from my mother, Marguerite (Peggy), whose voice you "hear" throughout in first-person form. Mother wanted you to know that; I said I didn't care and didn't think you would, either. I didn't want to detract from the story by volunteering that information up front, so we compromised and put it here in the back of the book, where you may or may not bother to read it.

When I began encouraging Mother to commit to paper her hard-won wisdom on the subject of caring for aging parents, she resisted. It was one thing, she said, to pass through that season; it was quite another to relive the adventure via paper and keyboard. Survival, for a time, was her most cherished souvenir, and she intended to relish the relief unencumbered.

"But you learned so much!" I persisted. "Don't you wish you'd had someone—a veteran like yourself, now—to offer some hope and a suggestion or two when your challenges began?"

Now *that* made her think. "I know what," she replied after a long moment, a Big Idea starting in her eye. (I've long since learned what that look means: work for me.) "Why don't *you* write a book? I'll help you figure out what to put in it. Of course, you witnessed firsthand most of what went on for those fourteen years; I probably don't have much to add. And you have such a way with words, my dear. So you write it, okay? Yes, let's do that," she concluded firmly, as if the matter were finished.

Well, somebody had to do it. There really was a story in the years she and Dad cared for her parents. I had been a witness to—and, at times, a participant in—the years of ministration to deserving forebears. Certainly I could tell the tale as well as almost anyone.

Or so I thought. This was one of those projects we begin with relative enthusiasm, certain that we have a contribution to make to the world, only to find (usually not far from the starting point) that ambition may exceed capacity. It's bad enough when we speak or perform for ourselves, but when, as in my case, the effort serves a far more deserving other (like my beloved mother), the Peter Principle[18] takes a scary twist. I may have exceeded my level of competence on this one, I reasoned, but I promised I'd complete the project. My honor was at stake. (For all her initial ambivalence, Mother got pretty excited about the whole idea after we'd discussed it for a couple of years.)

Add to that the fact that I told almost everyone I knew I was writing a book. I even took time off from work to finish. There was simply nowhere to go but through with it.

Let me conclude what I had hoped would be briefer remarks from the ghostdaughterwriter[19] with an observation. As I worked on this project, I interviewed a number of subjects, mostly informally. I was amazed that nearly everyone I spoke with, even casually, had at least a friend—and, more often, a close relative—undergoing a similar challenge with the next generation up. Few could report the same quality of relationship my mother had enjoyed with her parents. I found my dear friend, Rachelle, for instance, huddled in her bed one day, trying to recover from bronchial pneumonia and a dislocated shoulder, while simultaneously managing a household *and* a cantankerous father who threatened to sue her and her hus-

---

[18] A term originally used in the literature of business and management which suggests that individuals in an organization often rise to the level of their incompetence.

[19] A strange but descriptive word of my own creation.

band if they followed through with their long-overdue plan to relocate him to a convalescent center. Amidst her sobs, Rachelle confessed that she and her father had always suffered from a troubled relationship, and the invitation she and her husband extended to him to share their home some months ago came in spite of her painful childhood memories. His current behavior was resulting in greater stress for the entire family, and Rachelle's physical condition deteriorated along with her emotional state almost by the moment. "What am I going to do?" she pleaded tearfully. "It's come down to him or me; only one of us is going to survive if we maintain the status quo."

Then there's Jennifer. I had invited her to review an initial draft of my manuscript, given our past professional collaborations and a rather skimpy awareness that she had been involved in the care of aging parents and in-laws. Her response: a politely scathing, three-page retort suggesting, in essence, that Mother and I board our happy little spaceship and return to planet Earth. "Caring for my parents was a *joy?*" Jennifer almost screamed, quoting a line from the manuscript. "Get real!"

Well, thanks to Rachelle and Jennifer—and many others who dared to tell it like it really was, for them—this book is slightly more objective than it might have been. At least, I tried to acknowledge throughout, in a variety of ways, that Mother's experience was not representative of every caregiving encounter. But I maintain that certain common elements remain, most notable of which, perhaps, is that *caregiving is hard.*

Even if your loved ones are angels en route to heaven.

Suggested Readings and Resources

About Caregiving, South Deerfield, MA: Channing L. Bete Co., Inc., 1988. (For a copy of this booklet, telephone (800) 628-7733 and request item number 37341.)

About Pain Management, a pamphlet published by Choice in Dying, 200 Varick St., New York, NY 10014. Telephone: (212) 366-5540.

Aging Is a Family Affair: A Guide to Quality Visiting Long-Term Care Facilities and You, by Wendy Thompson, Toronto: NC Press, Ltd., 1987.

American Federation of Home Health Agencies, Silver Spring, MD. Telephone: (301) 588-1454.

The Caregiver's Guide: Helping Elderly Relatives Cope with Health and Safety Problems, by Caroline Rob and Janet Reynolds, Boston, MA: Houghton Mifflin Co., 1991.

Caregiving: How to Care for Your Elderly Mother and Stay Sane, by E. Jane Mall, New York, NY: Ballantine Books, 1990.

Caregiving: When Someone You Love Grows Old, by John Gillies, Wheaton, IL: H. Shaw Publishers, 1988.

Caring for Your Aging Parents: A Sourcebook of Timesaving Techniques and Tips, by Kerri S. Smith, Lakewood, CO: American Source Books, 1992.

The Challenge of Age: A Guide to Growing Older in Health and Happiness, by E. Fritz Schmerl and Sally Petterson Tubach, New York, NY: Continuum, 1986.

Coming Home: A Guide to Home Care for the Terminally Ill, by Deborah Duda, Santa Fe, NM: John Muir Publications, Inc., 1984.

Consumer Guide to Hospice Care, a booklet published by National Consumers League, 815 15th St., NW, Suite 928, Washington, D.C. 20005. Telephone: (202) 639-8140.

Eat More, Weigh Less, by Dean Ornish, New York, NY: HarperCollins Publishers, Inc., 1993.

Elder Care, a toll-free hotline for information regarding caregiving and support services in your area. Telephone: (800) 677-1116.

Gift from the Sea, by Anne Morrow Lindbergh, New York, NY: Vintage Books, 1978.

Guide to Choosing a Nursing Home, a free pamphlet from the U.S. Department of Health and Human Services, Health Care Financing Administration, 6325 Security Boulevard, Baltimore, MD 21207. (Request publication number HCFA-02174.)

Guide to Housing Alternatives for Older Citizens, by Margaret Gold, Mount Vernon, NY: Consumers Union, 1985.

A Handbook of Practical Care for the Frail Elderly, by Merlin A. Taber, Mary Ann Anichini, Steve Anderson, Robert A. Weagent, and the Community Care Project, University of Illinois School of Social Work, Phoenix, AZ: Oryx Press, 1986.

Healthy Older People, a free booklet available from the National Health Information Center, U.S. Department of Health and Human Services, P.O. Box 1133, Washington, DC 20012. Telephone: (800) 336-4797.

Helping Yourself Help Others, by Rosalynn Carter with Susan K. Golant, New York, NY: Random House, Inc., 1994.

Home Care Nursing: A Quick Reference Guide, by Carolyn J. Humphrey, Frederick, MD: Aspen Publishers, Inc., 1994.

If You're Over 65 and Feeling Depressed, a free booklet published by the National Institute of Mental Health. Telephone: (800) 421-4211.

Megahealth, by Marc Sorenson, Ivins, UT, 1992.

Miles Away and Still Caring (a guide to long-distance caregiving), American Association of Retired Persons, 601 E St. NW, Washington, DC 20049. Telephone: (202) 434-2277.

Modern Maturity, American Association of Retired Persons, 3200 E. Carson St., Lakewood, CA 90712.

National Association of Geriatric Case Managers, 655 N. Alvernon Way, Ste. 108, Tucson, AZ 85711. Telephone: (602) 881-8008.

National Hospice Organization, 1901 North Moore St., Suite 901, Arlington, VA 22209. Telephone: (800) 658-8898.

New Choices, Retirement Living Publishing Co., Inc., 28 W. 23rd St., New York, NY 10010.

The Other Generation Gap: The Middle Aged and Their Aging Parents, by Stephen Z. Cohen and Bruce Michael Gans, Chicago, IL: Follett Publishing Co., 1978.

Parenting Mom and Dad: A Guide for the Grown-up Children of Aging Parents, by Michael T. Levy, New York, NY: Prentice-Hall Press, 1991.

The Power of Optimism, by Alan Loy McGinnis, San Francisco, CA: Harper & Row, 1990.

We've Got to Do Something about Mother: Eleven Accounts of How Individuals Found Solutions to the Problem of Caring for Aging Parents, by Marilyn Richardson and J. Ryan Richardson, Brookings, SD: UniPress, 1990.

When Love Gets Tough: The Nursing Home Decision, by Doug Manning, Hereford, TX: Insight Books, Inc., 1983.

When Parents Age: What Children Can Do, by Tom Adams and Kathryn Armstrong, New York, NY: The Berkley Publishing Group, 1993.

When Your Parents Grow Old: Information and Resources to Help the Adult Son or Daughter Cope with the Problems of Aging Parents, by Jane Otten and Florence D. Shelley, New York, NY: Funk & Wagnalls, 1976.

You and Your Aging Parents: The Modern Family's Guide to Emotional, Physical, and Financial Problems, by Barbara Silverstone and Helen Kandel Hyman, New York, NY: Pantheon Books, 1976.

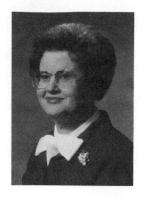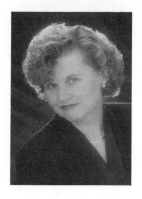

ABOUT THE AUTHORS

Marguerite Mauss Eliason was born in Salt Lake City, Utah, and raised in Oakland, California. She studied music and Japanese at the University of Puget Sound, although her first and most influential training was received from her mother, a renowned musician and teacher. She served an LDS mission in Japan, where she met her future husband, LeGrande Eliason, a fellow missionary. LeGrande and Marguerite have two daughters and three grandchildren. Their daughters' middle names—Chieko and Emiko—are evidence of their love for Japan and its people.

Susan Eliason holds a master's degree in organizational behavior and is currently employed as an instructional developer at the Missionary Training Center in Provo, Utah. She has designed and presented numerous management training programs in the U.S., Japan, and South Korea, and enjoys freelance writing and public speaking. She co-authored *Getting What You Want in Life without Feeling Guilty*.

Like her grandparents, parents, and her sister, Susan served an LDS mission in Japan. She is currently serving as a stake Relief Society president in a BYU stake.